Homeopathy

Strategies to Benefit From Homeopathic Medicine

(The Complete Guide to Treatment of Common Disorders)

David White

I0222733

Published By **Elena Holly**

David White

Homeopathy: Strategies to Benefit From Homeopathic Medicine (The Complete Guide to Treatment of Common Disorders)

ISBN   978-1-77485-773-1

Legal & Disclaimer

The information contained in this ebook is not designed to replace or take the place of any form of medicine or professional medical advice. The information in this ebook has been provided for educational & entertainment purposes only.

The information contained in this book has been compiled from sources deemed reliable, and it is accurate to the best of the Author's knowledge; however, the Author cannot guarantee its accuracy and validity and cannot be held liable for any errors or omissions. Changes are periodically made to this book. You must consult your doctor or get professional medical advice before using any of the suggested remedies, techniques, or information in this book.

Upon using the information contained in this book, you agree to hold harmless the Author from and against any damages, costs, and expenses, including any legal fees potentially resulting from the application of any of the

TABLE OF CONTENTS

Chapter 1: What's Homeopathy?

It is an all-encompassing approach to healing that provides the patient by using substances that are diminished. Most often, the drugs are given in tablets and are designed to activate an internal healing mechanisms. In essence, homeopathic practitioners rely on the notion that the body is able to heal itself, but it requires a bit of encouragement to make it happen in the case of more serious health conditions.

Although Homeopathic remedies are extremely beneficial to people, there are a few limitations to keep in mind while making use of these remedies. The best Homeopathic remedy usually requires advice of a qualified practitioner, who will give you the chance to get the most benefit from the treatment. It may take time, since the physician will need to offer you the correct combination of ingredients in order to determine the primary source of the issue can be addressed. There aren't any cure-all medicines and your doctor is required to provide you with a customized mix for your specific problems. So, don't believe that your medical issues will disappear overnight, since finding the most appropriate method of treatment will be a lengthy process.

If, for instance, you have a stomach pain that lasts for a long time the doctor will need to identify the root of the issue and the kind of ache it's and what's causing it worse, and any other symptoms you might be experiencing that might not be related. They'll then need to decide which treatment will be the most effective, and what dosage is most appropriate, based on various variables, such as your weight, age as well as the seriousness of the issue.

Homeopathic remedies are created by pharmacists who are experts in the preparation of the preparation of these weak chemicals. Utilizing a specific method (which will be discussed in the next chapter of the book) they develop an extremely specific formula to treat the condition you are suffering from. Although research hasn't yet been able of proving the exact way Homeopathy can benefit your health, and how it's remedies work within the body, it has been proven that these remedies have a positive effect on certain biological processes.

Many believe that the magic behind Homeopathic remedies lies in the brand new property created during the process of creation. When the remedies are being made, it's believed that there is an interaction between the substance that was originally used (such like the herb being utilized) and the ingredient is mixed with it (such like alcohol or water). In the course due to this interplay, a brand new structure is created which acts like the "active component" and remains in the mix, even when it gets diluted repeatedly.

The History of Homeopathy

It is believed that the first Practitioner of Homeopathy was Hippocrates who lived from 460 until 377 BC. Although he didn't use the Homeopathic remedies in use today but he did propose that like could treat like and that is one of the key principles of Homeopathy (which we'll talk about in the future in the book). A few centuries later, Paracelsus, a 16th century scientist who is called a pioneer in pharmaceutical science, believed that chemicals that cause a person to fall ill could be cured if they are taken in small amounts.

However, the Homeopathy we have is used today has been around for over two centuries. The "modern" form was developed in the late 18th century by Samuel Hahnemann, a German physician who was disgusted by the medical procedures that were practiced in the past that included bloodletting, the use of arsenic, poisons and even poisons. He began to look for new methods to lessen the negative consequences that are often associated with treatments for medical conditions. In the end, Dr. Hahnemann began to experiment with himself and a group of volunteers, by administering smaller doses of the most commonly used drugs. The doctor. Hahnemann discovered that these drugs were more effective and less harmful for the patient. He also observed that the negative side effects that occur as the result of toxic medication were similar to symptoms of the illnesses they were intended to treat.

"Dr. Hahnemann was also the person who invented"Homeopathy," which is also the name that was coined by Dr. Hahne "Homeopathy" by using the terms "homoios" (which is a synonym for like to similar in

Greek) in addition to "pathos" (which means suffering). It was founded on the "law of similar" principle that I will speak on in the following chapter. Homeopathy was very popular in the 19th century, just when The doctor Dr. Hahnemann began spreading the information about the advantages associated with Homeopathic remedies. The religious elite, literary legends as well as royalty started making use of these remedies in order to boost their health and heal diseases.

In the 1800s, a few students of Dr. Hahnemann's students established the first homeopathic school located in the United States. At the time, ailments like Scarlet Fever and Typhoid were widely spread and it was discovered that some remedies from Homeopathy were being utilized to treat these illnesses that could be life-threatening. In the early 1900s, some of the most famous universities were starting to offer Homeopathy instruction, like Stanford University and Boston University. There were also plenty of private Homeopathy schools which opened at this time.

In the 1920s The American Medical Association's opposition to alternative medicine as well as the advent of easy-to-use drugs reduced the demand for Homeopathic remedies across the Western world. However the usage of Homeopathy was growing steadily throughout Europe and Asia at the time. Due to the resurgence of holistic health and natural remedies, Homeopathy is becoming popular again, as more and more are starting to re-discover the advantages of Homeopathic remedies once more.

Homeopathy: The Principles of Homeopathy

There are three fundamental principles that are associated with Homeopathy and every remedy which are prescribed adheres to these basic theories:

Like cures like. Homeopathy is heavily based on the notion it is possible to treat similar with similar. For instance, if you are suffering from insomnia, you should consider a remedy from Homeopathy that is known to cause insomnia, like one that has caffeine can help you achieve an easier sleep. This is based on the idea that a substance that triggers certain symptoms could be dilute and then used in a remedy which can help treat the same symptoms.

Like cures like is commonly referred to as"law of similar. "law that applies to similar." In other words, when a person who is healthy is exposed to a certain substance and suffers symptoms or adverse effects then a remedy that contains the same ingredient can aid sufferers with the symptoms (even when they're not suffering from the disease that the remedy was created to treat). For example when a person is suffering from allergies , which include symptoms such as watery eyes and nasal congestion it is possible to prescribe an remedy that is made up of red onion. This is because onion's active ingredient could cause the same effects. Think of the time when you last cut an onion. You're likely to have suffered from watery eyes or running nose. So, as per Homeopathy it is possible to treat similar symptoms using the potentized onion regardless of whether the problem or illness is not caused by onions.

Give the minimum dose. It is recommended that the Homeopathic remedy should be as dilute as it is. In general, the remedy given will be extremely dilute in order for you to enjoy the effects of the drug without the adverse consequences. This is a particular rule that follows the principle of "potentization" which all homeopathic remedies have to follow. Potentization is typically quite complicated and requires several steps to create the most effective possible remedy.

Potentization allows patients to reap huge benefits from a lower dose of a substance. This also allows them to take these supplements without worrying about risks, since the process of dilution eliminates all the toxic chemicals that is present in the original substance. Additionally, this method allows patients to treat or cure illnesses with substances that might not be suitable to consume.

Do not rely on a single remedy. Whatever symptoms you're experiencing, you'll be offered only one treatment. The one remedy is intended to address the root of the issue and all the symptoms. This is quite different from the method by how traditional medical professionals deal with diseases currently. For instance, if you seek a general physician for a condition that exhibits multiple symptoms, you may likely be given a different medicine for each symptom. But an Homeopathic practitioner will offer you only one treatment that can be employed to treat all the symptoms that accompany the illness as well as the cause of the issue itself.

Treatment of conditions by Homeopathic remedies

Homeopathy is a great option for treating a array of medical issues. Here are a few most frequent health issues which Homeopathy remedies can aid in relieving.

Digestive Issues. Homeopathy is a method to treat a variety of digestive disorders, including constipation, diarrhea, gas and heartburn, gastric reflux duodenal ulcers, hemorrhoids and anal fissures IBS (IBS) as well as Crohn's Disease. It is also utilized to treat polyps in the digestive tract. For instance, if you are suffering from rapid diarrhea, your physician might suggest phosphorous when diarrhea that is caused by nausea may require an Ipecac-based homeopathic treatment.

Infections. Croup is a common cold. influenza, fever tonsillitis, ear infections impetigo, bronchitis, coughs ringsworm, cold sores and impetigo are all instances of infections which can be treated using Homeopathy.

Headaches and migraines. People who have chronic headaches or migraines could get relief from a homeopathic remedy. The kind of headache but, will decide which treatment is recommended. Stress-related headaches require Ignatia as headaches resulting by mental stress requires Ruta Grav. Headaches are an excellent illustration of how the various types of an ailment could significantly alter the treatment options for the remedy that is homeopathic. There are remedies specifically designed to aid sufferers of headache caused from sitting in the sun over a long period of time, or wearing things on your head that is too tight, or headaches that are more severe in the evening. Each of these situations requires the use of a specific treatment.

Emotional Issues (depression anxiety, depression, etc.). Anxiety, mental haze poor memory as well as panic disorder and panic attacks Irrational fear (phobias), OCD (obsessive compulsive disorder), PTSD (post-traumatic stress disorder) and a myriad of other mental and emotional issues can be treated with homeopathic remedies.

Chronic Pain (general sciatica, back pain Sciatica, general back pain, etc.). Chronic back pain joint and muscle pain, as well as sciatica are all instances of pain which can be relieved with Homeopathy. Osteoarthritis, Rheumatoid Arthritis, frozen shoulder, tendinitis and osteoporosis patients are patients of chronic pain, and could benefit from homeopathic treatments.

Allergies. A lot of people sufferers of chronic allergies are troubled by the notion that non-prescription allergy remedies, or even the ones prescribed by traditional medical professionals are ineffective. Indeed, those suffering from allergies frequently find that not only the medications do not have any effects on the symptoms of allergy like a watery eyes and runny nose and swollen eyes, but they also result in adverse negative effects. Homeopathic remedies can provide relief from allergies by strengthening your system of the body so that it is able to fight off allergens causing the symptoms. Instead of treating the symptoms the remedies of Homeopathy actually strengthen your body's immune system , and activate your body's natural defense system in order to provide it with the ability to protect your body from harmful allergens.

ADHD/ADD. Homeopathy is a method for treating ADD (attention deficit) by treating the symptoms of the disease instead of trying to treat the condition in itself. In the end, symptoms that are present can be reduced and future problems could be prevented completely. The homeopathic treatment to treat ADHD and ADD includes 2 steps: Natural remedies and psychotherapy.

Hypertension of the Blood (Hypertension). Homeopathy is a great remedy for problems with blood pressure, for example, low or high blood pressure. Certain treatments are recognized to aid in balancing the levels of cholesterol in the body.

Infant Concerns. Common issues that can arise in infants can be addressed by Homeopathy for colic, cradle cap jaundice, thrush, reflux teething, skin eruptions.

Bladder Infections. Bladder infections and urinary tract infections and interstitial cystitis all can be treated with appropriate dosages of homeopathic treatments.

Sleeping Disorders. If you're experiencing trouble getting to sleep at night, Homeopathy may be able to aid you. Sleepless nights, chronic snoring and sleep apnoea as well as sleepwalking and insomnia are frequent sleep disorders that can be addressed as well as restless leg syndrome as well as night terrors.

Women's health issues. Menstrual disorders, menopausal concerns PMS, hot flashes are all addressed with custom-made Homeopathic treatments that are recommended by a certified Naturopath.

Skin Problems. Topical treatments made of homeopathic remedies are usually extremely effective when used to treat skin issues. The issues that could be addressed or even eliminated completely include acne, psoriasis abscesses, wartsand hives ulcers, Candida as well as various other fungal ailments.

Men's Health Issues. Erectile dysfunction, prostate issues and a decrease in sexual libido are common issues for males that could be addressed with an herbal treatment.

Infertility/Pregnancy Issues. If you are suffering from problems with infertility related to fibroids, endometriosis, poly-cystic-ovarian syndrome could discover that homeopathic remedies could assist. This holistic healing method is a great option to treat the issues that arise due to the pregnancy (such as morning nausea, aching veins and hemorrhoids) as well as breast feeding issues (lactation). It also helps help the mom prepare for the birth.

Chapter 2: What Are Homeopathic Remedies

Produced?

You may be thinking about the process by which Homeopathic remedies are derived by combining various flowers and plants that are collected to use for medicinal purposes. If you've ever visited an health food store you've likely seen numerous Homeopathic remedies that are available in various forms, like tablets and pills as well as creams and lotions. What is the process for converting flowers into pill form? The method is different based on the remedy as well as the origin of the remedy obtained. There are a variety of herbs minerals, plants, and other substances are utilized to make extremely powerful Homeopathic remedies. The method is usually the same for all makers however, some may opt to utilize an alternative diluting solution. Alcohol is the most common solution, however there are various preference based on the manufacturer. If you're making your own recipe alcohol, vodka or rum could be utilized. Any alcohol that is at least 80-100 proof is suitable Some even opt to make use of brandy.

Making an Mother Tincture

Since the majority of Homeopathic remedies originate from plants There is a method which must be followed to extract the beneficial ingredients and healing chemicals out of the plants. The first step of the process of making Homeopathic medicines is known as making your mother tincture.

The plant is macerated or softened by water. This is done through placing it in boiling water or the plant being allowed to soak in the water that has been heated by the sun for around three hours. The more woody plants are usually created using this method of boiling the water, whereas flowers heads that are softer are macerated with the latter. Certain methods require the mix of the water with alcohol throughout the process. Other methods include the alcohol only after the plant is soaked. After the proper amount of time for soaking the mixture is then squeezed to get rid of the plant particles. What remains are the chemicals that you want to remove that are extracted from the plant. This solution is known by the name of the Mother Tincture. It will be utilized to achieve the desired strength at the following step.

Potentiation via Succussion

In order to create a remedy succussion-potentiation. A drop of mother tincture is added to an vial. If you are doing this at home use a mason jar fitted with lid can be used. Based on the strength you want of the solution, a specific quantity of alcohol-water solution are added. A typical mix comprises one drop of the mother tincture, and nine drops of mixture of water and alcohol.

The next step is essential in the process. The vial should be shaken vigorously in order to blend the mother tincture and the water and alcohol solution. This can be accomplished by placing a stopper in the vial, and then pounding on a table, desk or any other solid surface. If you use one drop of the mother tincture, and 9 drops of solution of water, the product will have the potency of 1x. To increase the strengthof the product, you'd need to go through the similar process using the same solution that was created from the initial sucussion process.

Potentiation through Trituration

Trituration is a process to remove the chemical from solid substances and can't be collected via succusion. Consider things like gold. However long you shake or soak it, you will not be able get any of the valuable chemicals from it! If you take for instance gold, the method of grinding could be employed. The mortar and the pestle can be used to crush the solid matter and make fine dust. The other substance is utilized in order to dissolve the material. For the gold mineral, sugar powder can be an excellent dilutizer. Depending on the nature of the material is, it undergoes this process until it is at either an 8x or 9x level of potency. This is when it's sufficiently fine to pass through the process of succussion, but it takes a lot of energy and effort for grinding the material into an extremely fine powder.

Liquids Gels, Creams Pellets, Tablets, or Liquids

The last step to create homeopathic remedies is deciding what the final format will be. There are many options available, and each remedy has the use of a specific final form depending on the purpose it is to be utilized for. Certain things aren't designed to be eaten and therefore require the form of gel or cream.

Liquids are the base form that all Homeopathic remedies begin. The liquid is then used to make the other types.

Liquids can be added to gels or creams for external use. Many lotions or essential oils may act as carriers for liquid homeopathic formulations. The majority of remedies are poisonous when applied directly to the skin. They are generally suggested to be mixed with an oil to apply to the wound or for use as an oil or salve.

Pellets are made of sugar or hard sucrose. The liquid solution is sprayed over sugar pellets that are hard. To prevent the sugar from dissolved the solution has to contain at least at 87 percent alcohol. The solution dissolves inside the mouth, and can be consumed orally. Avoid touching the pellet to prevent the remedy from melting on your hands rather than inside the mouth.

Tablets are similar to the ones you buy however they are manufactured using easily dissolvable lactose or milk sugar. These are small white pills with the Homeopathic solution in the tablets before being solidified. As a result, it is safe to rub the tablets.

They're taken in similarly to pellets and it is suggested that they be put under the tongue for rapid absorption into the body.

What Homeopathic constitutional type are you?

Every patient who goes to a practitioner of Homeopathy falls within any of these "constitutional" types. The types of Constitution will be determined by a myriad of factors, such as the patient's present emotional and mental state, the physical appearance, what kind of clothes he wears and also whether they prefer to be in a private setting or with an environment with others. The ability to determine your constitutional type can allow Naturopaths to provide the most effective treatments since this allows them to pinpoint the remedies that are most appropriate to a specific type of emotion. For instance, if, for example, there are four options for tension headaches and the fourth option is most appropriate for the person's specific constitution and type, then that is the one generally recommended.

Below is an outline of fifteen Common Constitutional Types to help you to figure out which one you might fall into. If you're not sure after reading this information, you might want to conduct further studies to find out which classification best fits your needs.

Argentum Nitricum. The types that look older than they are This is usually caused by stress and worry. They also have pale skin and are always on the move. They can experience nervous sweats as well as nerve system weakness and mucous membranes that are weak. People in this category tend to be extroverted and anxious. They like salty and sweet food however, they prefer hot food in preference to those served cold.

Arsenicum Album. These are usually thin and feature delicate appearances. They also have sensitive skin that is prone to wrinkles. The main weaknesses are located in the heart, the skin and liver as well as stomach. They are often afflicted by digestive problems. They are extroverts and can be described as perfectionists. They enjoy sweet and sour dishes and fatty foods (such as junk food) as well as coffee.

Calcium Carbonicum. They are usually obese and slow-moving. They are often overweight and tired. They're sensitive and impressionable and tend to be calm. They usually require the motivation to be successful and encouragement from other people. The weaknesses they suffer from are in the ear, nose and throat, and inside the bones. They could also be susceptible to digestive issues. They are fond of milk products and carbohydrates as well as cold foods.

Graphite. They are usually overweight. They generally have a rough appearance that is dry and has rough appearance. They have a reputation for taking their time to tackle problems they encounter, and possess the capacity to focus intensely on one task at a time. They're not morning people, and tend to have mood fluctuations. Their biggest weaknesses lie in their nails and skin. They can also be afflicted with fatigue and nosebleeds. They are more prone to sour and savory food items.

Ignatia. They are slim and frequently have dark circles under their eyes. They appear tired all the time and sometimes display facial movements. They're extremely strung and have extreme mood swings. They are also noted for their dependency on smoking and caffeine. Their weaknesses are related to the nervous system and they may suffer from emotional issues. This is why they can suffer from frequent migraines, colds, the twitching of their hands, and constipation. They are drawn to savory and sour food items, and also dairy products.

Lachesis. The people who suffer from it usually have an unchanging expression and tend to be slim. They generally have pale skin and strong eyes. The most well-known features of this type of person is that they tend to lick their lips often. They tend to be optimistic, but their thoughts may become scattered. They are also very talkative. Their weaknesses include issues with circulation, varicose veins, as well as menopausal concerns. They may also be suffering from insomnia. They are fond of alcohol, coffee and cool drinks in addition to food items that are sour and sweet.

Lycopodium. They tend to be slim and show visible lines of worry on their faces. They generally appear older than they really are. They may also be suffering from visible facial movements. They are famous for their drama.

They they are also anxious and shy about engagement. They also are afraid of being lonely. For the weaknesses they have, they typically have digestive issues as well as sore throats along with the chronic fatigue syndrome. They love sweets and warm beverages, but no flavored meats.

Mercurius Solubilis. Patients who suffer from this condition sweat frequently and appear radiant. They struggle with their emotions and aren't able to believe in people easily. They don't handle criticism well, and are notorious for their memory issues. They usually experience exhausted, sore throats sensitized skin and seasonal Affective Disorder. They love carbs, cold drinks and have a special love of citrus fruits.

Natrium Muriatricum. The people who suffer from this condition are slim and strong and are pear-shaped (if they're female). The skin of these individuals is often unnaturally puffy, and they usually have eyes that are red. They hide their emotions , and frequently have depression because of it. They have a difficult time dealing with breaking up and are focused on their work. Their weaknesses are related to the nervous system such as anorexia, headaches, and anorexia. They are averse to cold food and drinks, and also spicy and sour foods.

Nux Vomica. The people who are Nux Vomica are thin and appear always tense. They get older prematurely and usually suffer from dark circles under their eyes. They are prone to developing addictions and can be prone to overindulge. They also are extremely anxious and are afraid of failure more than everything other things. They are susceptible to digestive problems, migraines headaches, hernias, and migraines. They are prone to fatty food as well as alcohol and coffee and spicy foods.

Phosphorus. They are thin and tall and are known to be fashionable. the latest fashions. They're also talented and require plenty of attention. They are fun to be around at a gathering as well as in group however, they can be demanding at certain times. They're also affectionate and don't hesitate of expressing their true emotions. They are susceptible to nervous system disorders as well as circulation issues and headaches. They like sour and sweet food items, carbonated drinks and alcohol.

Pulsatilla. The people who suffer from this condition are often overweight, but they're usually pretty. They have a beautiful complexion and are often confused with younger people. They're shy, gentle and never confident. They do not like confrontation, and may suffer from obsessive compulsive behavior. They are susceptible to reproductive issues in females, Irritable Bowel Syndrome, and varicose veins. They like sweet as well as cold food.

Sepia. They are slim and tall and prefer sitting in a cross-legged position. They are usually elegant and polished. They can easily be offended and don't want to be around crowds. They have strong opinions and aren't afraid of communicate them to others. They are susceptible to headaches, menopausal symptoms and skin problems as well as the chronic fatigue syndrome. They are fond of sour and savory food items, sweet and citrus.

Silica. Silica is a thin type with big foreheads. In reality, it appears that their heads are too large in comparison to their physique. They are beautiful and their hands tend to sweat. They have low self-confidence and often feel exhausted mentally. They're indecisive and be overwhelmed in a short time. They are known for their fear of failing. They are susceptible to issues with the nervous system fatigue, exhaustion and respiratory issues and headaches. They are averse to cold food and stay clear of hot food items.

Sulphur. These kinds of people are usually slim and have a poor posture. They are often unclean and also have lips and skin that are red. Their minds are typically overflowing with thoughts, and they are known to engage in arguments with other people. They have low self-esteem and are often criticized for their inability to complete tasks. They are susceptible to constipation and skin problems as well as issues with body odor. They are prone to consuming fat-rich and sweet food items, and also alcohol.

Chapter 3: Beginning To Get Started With

Homeopathy

This section will provide all the details that you need to start in the field of Homeopathy at your own pace (if you've not had the opportunity to meet with an expert in Homeopathy or develop your own treatment program to improve your overall health). While I'd suggest consulting with an Homeopathic specialist if you are planning to utilize Homeopathic remedies however, there are certain instances in which you are capable of purchasing ready-made remedies from health food stores that could offer you a wealth of advantages.

Remember, if intend to treat yourself with Homeopathic remedies, make sure you purchase your medicines from reputable sellers. If you're suffering from a serious medical issue or your illness is getting worse it is recommended that you seek help from a qualified health professional whenever you can.

In the beginning of your journey into the realm of Homeopathy It is highly recommended to use only a couple of remedies for the first time. Explore them thoroughly and conduct a great deal of research prior to that to find out the benefits they provide, and whether they can provide relief from the symptoms you are experiencing. If, for instance, you're thinking of making use of a particular remedy that addresses a range of symptoms (including ones you don't have) You might be interested in looking at other remedies that are less specific in its range of symptoms that can be treated.

To identify the exact symptoms you're experiencing be sure to monitor your health over the duration throughout the entire day. This might seem like a strange task. You are the best at identifying your body's needs and you are likely to be aware of the aches and discomforts you experience regularly. You might be amazed by the number of the aches and aches are just something we get used to (until you don't feel them anymore). Therefore, I highly recommend you to spend the day taking note of the signs of something wrong within your body, to find the remedy from homeopathy that is most appropriate to your specific needs and ailments.

A second important thing to do is be aware of the way your body reacts to different stimuli or triggers. For instance how do you react to stress caused by being sick? Do things like sudden movement and the heat of your room aggravating the symptoms you're experiencing? These factors can assist you to determine the best treatment.

Once you've compiled the list of symptoms, it's now time to pick a solution. In this process, be sure that you choose a remedy that will best suit your specific needs. The majority of products that are available include explicit descriptions of what they are able to treat, including specific medical conditions as well specific symptoms. If you're able to identify the remedy that works for your specific condition and needs and the remedies' actions mirror your own reaction to the illness, ailment or stress you're experiencing. In this way, it will provide you with the capability to trigger your own defense mechanism and address the issues that are causing destruction in your overall health wellbeing.

It is recommended to take only an amount of remedy that you've selected, and then watch to see how you respond to the remedy. If you observe the symptoms diminishing or gone, you're sure that the remedy is effective. Do not take another dose of the Homeopathic treatment if it's effective, since this could reduce its effectiveness. You should not do it until you realize the improvement in your overall health has ceased.

It's crucial to remember that homeopathic dosage doesn't follow a predetermined timetable. In essence you must apply the remedy when you notice that your body ceases reacting to it. If you're experiencing an immediate or painful issue, you might need to take larger doses of. If you're suffering from severe pain, I would suggest you consult a medical expert immediately. While some treatments like those designed to ease headaches might require administration several times per hour, other remedies, such as the ones used to treat a cold might only have to be taken a couple of times per day.

If you try the medication and don't see any changes, you might prefer to wait a little longer before giving another dose. If you do not notice any improvements after several doses, it is recommended to review your symptoms to determine which remedy is best for your health requirements. It could be that the method you've chosen isn't suitable for your specific type of symptoms and another remedy similar to it could be better suited.

If you are self-medicating Homeopathic remedies, low potencies tend to be the most effective. This is due to the fact that higher doses may be more effective and more rapid in their action however the choice of remedies should be more specific. It may be beneficial to begin with a potency of 6X instead of a 30 C (C scale). Anything higher than a 30 C should only be used by experienced Homeopathic professionals. If you're not seeing any change in your symptoms even after many attempts at a remedy (or maybe after using a few similar remedies) You may need to seek out a professional who is qualified.

The Homeopathic remedy list and their applications

Sulphur

Sulphur is among the most well-known Homeopathic remedies because of its numerous uses when it is combined with other ingredients from Homeopathy. It is, by itself, used to treat various skin conditions. Inflammation, redness, and scaling that are caused by eczema, or other rashes have been treated by sulphur for about 2000 years. The properties of sulphur are strong and have been utilized successfully to treat a variety of ailments listed below:

The physical and emotional signs of premenstrual symptoms

- Nightmares

- Indecisiveness or listlessness

- Used to build determination and drive

- Digestive aid, nausea, vomiting, and digestion

Back pain is due to sitting too much

- Migraines

Respiratory infections that cause either yellow or green sputum

- Eye infections

Arsenicum Album

It is derived from arsenic which naturally occurs in the soil, arsenicum can be utilized to treat a range of illnesses in a safe way. It can be consumed as a pill that dissolves, in powder form or that dissolves in liquid. It is believed to be among the top 15 remedies of the first aid kit of Homeopathic remedies because of its capacity to treat various diseases. One of the most controversial applications of arsenicum album can be as a tonic treatment for arsenic poisoning based upon the Homeopathic Law of Similars. Apart from that it is frequently employed to treat more typical ailments of the body:

- Chills, flu symptoms as well as fever, anxiety

skin conditions such as the scalp flaky, psoriasis or dry eczema

- Indigestion, heartburn

- Anxiety

- Colds can cause an odour that is watery from the nose or respiratory problems

Eyes that are itchy or watery, itchy and red

- Asthma

- Diarrhea

Phosphorus

Phosphorus is an naturally occurring mineral found in the human body and is vital for a healthy body as well as mind. It helps in the function of cells and has been extensively used as a component of Homeopathic and traditional medicines. It is regarded as one of the most beneficial ingredients in the treatment of a range of mental and physical ailments:

- Respiratory issues, difficulty breathing, chest pain.

It is used to treat the adverse effects of food poisoning

- Gum bleeding and chronic nosebleeds

A feeling of burning pain throughout the body

- Fear and anxiety

Eye problems, such as blurred vision, or problems arising due to cataracts

Calcarea Carbonica

Calcarea carbonica is one of the most common remedies component of the Homeopathic medicine kit. It is utilized as a treatment for constitution rather than for specific symptoms. In essence, this means that all symptoms are examined together with their medical and genetic background. The Constitutional therapy is intended to treat a chronic illness or issue. It is among the three major Homeopathic treatments that is often targeted towards the skin and irritants. When it is used in conjunction with other Homeopathic remedies, it is also utilized to treat the following conditions:

Symptoms that get worse in colder conditions

Teething

Ulcers

- Gallstones

- Bronchitis

- Asthma

Blood pressure : High

Lycopodium Clavatum

This Homeopathic remedy is used since the 1800s to treat digestive stimulant and appetite stimulant. It is the result of an evergreen plant that is commonly utilized to treat stomach issues however, it has been highly effective in treating eczema. It is commonly known as Club Moss, Fox Tail or Lamb's Tail. Wolf's Claw. The spores from the plants have been utilized for many years to treat gout and treat wounds. If taken internally, it helps to treat digestion issues, and also treats:

- Urine retention

- Bloating

Prostate or kidney issues

- Infections of the chest

Headache

- Vomiting, nausea

- Constipation

Hemorrhoids that are bleeding

- Insomnia

- Anxiety

Pulsatilla Nigricans

Also known as wind-flower Pulsatilla nigricans is an excellent remedy to keep around. It is extremely versatile. In the early days of Homeopathy it was utilized to treat eye ulcers as well as inflammations. Today, it's been proven to be effective in treating a range of illnesses including:

- Backaches

- Bed-wetting (only in the event of a child being sick)

Common cold, with green or yellow nasal discharge

Dry cough

- Diarrhea

- Eye inflammation

- Joint pain

- Teething/toothache

- Varicose veins

Graphite

Pure graphite that is ground into powder is often utilized as a homeopathic treatment. This mineral is extracted from carbon, and it has potent healing properties. Like many Homeopathic treatments graphite is a great choice to treat skin eruptions. In fact, this was the way it was first found. Employees of a mirror manufacturing facility used graphite to treat their cold sores. It did the trick! Since then, there's been further discoveries in the field of using graphite for treating a variety of conditions:

- Eczema that bleeds.

- Dry, cracked skin

- Psoriasis

Infected cuts can cause infection

Scratchy marks

- Hair loss

Ulcers

Menstrual flow is irregular or absent. flow

- Digestive disorders that cause gas and bloating that is painful, as well as gas.

- Aversions to people or shyness

Sepia

Sepia is derived from cuttlefish which are found on the Mediterranean Sea, and it is usually associated with artistic uses. However it is also used within Homeopathy this is an popular treatment for women's problems. It has proven to be to be effective in treating the adverse effects of the premenstrual cycle as well as hot flashes caused due to menopausal symptoms. Sepia can be utilized to treat more than treating issues relating to feminine reproductive system. It is usually included in regular Homeopathic first-aid kits due to its broad spectrum of use. It has been proven to be efficient in treating:

- Lactation difficulties after the birth

Constipation

- Hemorrhoids

Indigestion that is caused through the consumption of dairy products

- Mucus triggered by allergies or cold

Abdominal tenderness is due to gas

- Circulatory disorders that cause sweating or chills.

Muscle pain and exhaustion

Rhus Toxicodendron

This is the best treatment to treat arthritis pain. It is anti-inflammatory which makes it beneficial to those suffering from joint swelling due to arthritis. The stiffness that gets worse when you move is also alleviated by Rhus tox. Alongside arthritis, this drug is also utilized to treat a variety of other diseases too:

Menstrual cycles that are heavy or long periods

Tingling and numbness arms or legs because of overexertion

Skin itching or burning eruptions

Herpes - Herpes

A muscle strain or strain that has been strained or strained

41

- Relieves the effects of Ivy or poison oak eruptions

Natrum Muriaticum

Natrum muriaticum is normally prepared by a homeopath practitioner through drinking down table salt, is a remedy that can help treat various physical and mental ailments. Salt is then absorbed by the body's tissues and is thought to be the cause of an individual's ailments.

It is also believed to improve your immune system. Women who are pregnant are frequently given Natrum Muriaticum to fight off the effects of toxemia during the final weeks of pregnancy. One of the primary uses of this remedy is treating mental illnesses like:

A lot of grief

Nightmares

- Phobias

- Constant sadness/depression

- Sensitivity

Mercurius Vivus

Mercurius vius is derived from mercuric chloride. However it is safe to use and doesn't have the same toxic properties like mercury. Contrary to most Homeopathic cures, this one isn't as widespread and is only employed to treat a few of issues. The most commonly used use of the mercurius vivus remedy is to treat stomach ulcers, specifically those that lead to diarrhea. Mundal ulcers are often treated using this treatment.

Belladonna

Belladonna can be described as a multiple-use drug that can treat a range of physical and mental conditions. It is important to note that excessive belladonna can be toxic and, like any medication, it is recommended to adhere to dosage guidelines. It comes from the deadly nightshade plant and in the in the past, its poisonous qualities were utilized as a weapon to kill. In Homeopathy concoctions, it's reduced in volume and is considered to be as safe. It is usually given to patients suffering from anxiety or nervousness because it aids in relaxation and has a calming effect. Other ailments it can be used for include

- Fever and swelling

- Symptoms that are related to the flu

Sunstroke - Sunstroke

Blood pressure : High

Causticum

It has been a long-standing solution to conditions that cause burning or intense pain. It's also proven to be to be effective in treating other chronic ailments, including carpal tunnel syndrome and also for:

- Sore throat and difficulty swallowing

Dry, deep cough that has no sputum was brought up

Urinary disorders, including bed-wetting

Warts that easily bleed

Tremors in the muscles and Bell's Palsy

The restless leg syndrome

- Fibromyalgia

Constipation

Nux Vomica

Nux vomica is frequently employed to treat a wide range of digestive disorders. Women who are pregnant often use the remedy to treat morning sickness. Problems caused by the digestive system, such as constipation, bloating, or diarrhea can be addressed by taking nux vomica. This remedy is typically reserved for those who have Type A personality types. The majority of digestive issues people experience could be related to their temperamental personality. That's why it is recommended to use nux vomica for treating this, as well as other conditions, including:

- Stomach cramps

- Insomnia

- Irritability

- Cough not related to the cold

Headache

Lachesis

Lachesis comes by the venom from a bushmaster that is found in South Africa. It is a fantastic treatment for circulatory issues since it's an healthy blood thinner. People who have blue extremities can use lachesis to improve circulation. Women with extreme premenstrual symptoms may utilize the remedy of Homeopathy to ease the symptoms. Lachesis is also utilized to treat:

- Chest pains

- Heartbeat irregularity

- Menopause

- Extreme throat pain

- Epileptic seizures

- Tremors resulting from weak muscles

Ulcers

Burns, Burns

Insect bites

Silicea

Silicea is a popular treatment for a variety of skin issues It can also be utilized to treat mood disorders too. Silicea is derived from quartz that naturally occurs or flint. It is found in human bodies in cartilage and bones. It is also used to treat various health issues, but most commonly used use is to enhance beauty. Nail, skin and hair issues are frequently treated using silicea, in addition to:

Acne - Acne

- Skin blemishes

Dry skin

- Nails with brittleness

- Anemia

- Vertigo

- Preventing dandruff

- Scars that heal

Nitricum Acidum

It is also known by the name nitric acids This Homeopathic remedy is commonly employed to treat a variety of skin issues. It's very like mercurius vivus however, it is usually prescribed to people with dark hair, while one mercurius vivus is for people with light hair. Other conditions that it treat include

Blisters or ulcers can be found on the tongue, or other regions of the mouth

The mouth can be irritated or a fissure may form around the mouth

Warts

- Hemorrhoids

- Anal fissures

Apis Mellifica

The remedy for Homeopathy is derived of bees, with stingers also included. After crushing, it is then fermented with alcohol it becomes a homeopathic remedy that is for treating swelling that can be caused by a variety of ailments, such as bites from insects and bees in addition to:

- Infections of the urinary tract

- Edema

Blisters

- Allergies that cause difficulty swallowing

- Pleurisy

Fevers

- Measles

Mumps

Nettle rash

Aconitum Napellus

It is an essential item in your Homeopathy medication cabinet. It's a quick cure to treat the symptoms of chills and fevers that are often related to the flu. Sniffles that are triggered by changing weather conditions can be treated using the aconitum napellus. The remedy should be taken in the initial stages of illness will ensure an immediate recovery. The remedy comes from the monkshood weed, and even though the plant makes an astringent that was previously employed as a dip for arrows, it also contains therapeutic properties. It is commonly used to treat:

- Symptoms of the flu and cold

Bladder infections

Headaches

Colic - Colic

Kreosotum

Kreosotum is often known as creosote. It is made of beechwood tar. It was in the past was used as a preservative for wood but only became known for its healing properties within the last few hundred years. Its applications haven't been explored to the fullest extent however, for the moment homeopathic physicians suggest it for treating:

- Bed-wetting issues

Teethache and decay

Women are at risk for yeast infections.

- Nausea during pregnancy

- Bleeding between menstrual cycles

Carbo Vegetabilis

This is the treatment that is recommended to people suffering from indigestion and heartburn. It is absorbed by the body, which can hinder stomach acid. Bloating and gastric discomfort is a common treatment. Like the majority of Homeopathic remedies, this one is multi-functional, and it is commonly employed to treat:

- Flu

Infections

- Mononucleosis

A rattling cough

Voice loss

- Weak digestion

Bryonia Alba

Byronia alba, also known as what people refer to as the white barony, because of the plant that the medicine made, is poisonous, and should not be consumed in the absence of proper preparation. In reality, it's this root which is prescribed by Homeopathic physicians to patients suffering from arthritis. Anti-inflammatory properties make this the most sought-after remedy for:

Achy joints, stiff joints result from swelling

Neck and back discomfort

- Sciatica

- Fibromyalgia

- Tendonitis

Agaricus Muscarius

Agaricus muscarius originates from a poisonous fungus that is well-known because of its vivid red cap. It is being used in children suffering from ADHD but is most frequently employed to treat twitching and spasms. Arthritis which causes spasms and jerking is treated using this method. The spinal problems that result in burning or involuntary jerking along the spine can also be treated using agaricus Muscarius. In addition, it's efficient in treating:

Alcohol withdrawal symptoms include shaking and shaking

Bell's Palsy

Argentum Nitricum

This is an essential solution for people suffering from anxiety. Patients who have taken the medication prior to speaking in public have reported feeling at ease , despite previous anxiety. The remedy is generally used to treat stage anxiety. It has been used to treat a number of digestive problems, like diarrhea.

Baryta Carbonica

It is often referred to by its name simply as Bar-C, the remedy is often used for older people and children who suffer from various illnesses. Children who are diagnosed as mentally retarded and could be suffering from growth delay are treated by using baryta carbonica. People with dementia or issues with mobility are treated using this, too. It is also employed to treat other ailments:

- Prostate enlargement

- Seizures

Muscles moving

Recurrent respiratory infections

- The recurrence of throat infections

- High cholesterol

Alumina

Alumina is a product of the mineral aluminium , and is usually employed as an anti-acid. Contrary to the aluminum used present in over-the-counter anti-acids Alumina is reduced enough that it is safe. Recent studies have revealed an alarming amount of aluminum found in the brains of people suffering from Alzheimer's. In addition to being an acid-reducing agent, it is also used for treating various other ailments like:

- Fatigue/exhaustion

- Dementia

- Appetite disorders

- Constipation

Kali Carbonicum

Kali carbonicum, composed of potassium carbonate is utilized to treat respiratory conditions which include asthma. The remedy is diluted enough to allow it to be taken internally. Practitioners often make an tincture or salve to rub into the skin in order to relieve joint and back pain and also:

- Relief from pain caused by kidney stones

- Insomnia

Conium Maculatum

The poisonous hemlock that is what the Homeopathic treatment conium maculatum taken from. In the past, in Greek times, hemlock was utilized to poison executions. However, thanks to an dilution process the remedy is safe and is able for treating a wide range of illnesses, including:

- Gland exaggerations of the Gland

- Vertigo

Headaches that result from the impact of a blow or falling

Eye problems caused by an injury to the eye.

Menopausal-related side effects

- Pain or difficulty when you urinate.

- Nervous disorders

Hepar Sulphuris Calc

It is a popular treatment for those suffering from acne. It has been proved to help clear the skin quickly. Skin eruptions that release pus can be treated using Hepar Sulph. Other issues it treats are:

Abscesses

- Dental infections

- Ear infections

Cough, either mucus-free or with

- Sore throat

- Styes on the eyes

Aurum Metallicum

The aurum metallicum supplement is known as the Prozac of homeopathic medicine. It is derived from precious metal gold. It is an effective mood booster. depression sadness, despair and other feelings of sadness can all be addressed with this treatment. When you experience traumatizing events that be a trigger for depression, doctors will usually suggest this powerful mood booster. While reducing depression is the most frequent application of this treatment however, there are a handful of other uses like:

- Improves blood circulation the blockages that can cause headaches.

- Breathing difficulty

Liver problems, such as jaundice and liver disease.

- Chest pains that are sporadic.

Mezereum

Mezereum is usually used as a treatment for many skin eruptions. Eczema, eczema and psoriasis are some of the most frequently treated conditions by mezereum. However, it could be suggested for someone who suffers from an ulcer or burning pains in the abdomen. Bone pain is also treated by this method.

Phosphoricum Acidum

This homeopathic medicine is utilized to treat emotional issues such as exhaustion and stress. It is basically dilute the phosphoric acid. Someone who is excessively overwhelmed or tired due to grieving will usually be advised to use phosphoricum acidum. The negative effects of exhaustion, such as the feeling of lethargy, confusion, and lack of energy, remembering, and lethargy - are all addressed by this treatment. It can also be used to treat:

Reduce the calcium levels of cancer patients

- Digestive stimulant

- Prevent hair loss

- Prevent diabetes

China Officinalis

China officinalis, also known as what many people who are who are knowledgeable about Homeopathy call simply China helps to relieve muscle spasms as well as cramping. It is derived from quinine bark. It is a multi-purpose treatment that is able to treat various health issues including:

- Lower back discomfort

Tingling and rigid toes feet

Indigestion; gas; and gas and

Stomachache

- Pain in the nerves

Headaches

Ringing or buzzing the ear

Meniere's Disease

Petroleum

The substance is coal oil. petroleum is a well-known treatment used in traditional medicine in jelly form. In Homeopathy it is dilute and then formulated into a pill to treat many ailments. For both conventional and Homeopathic medical practices the use of petroleum is for treating skin problems that cause cracked or dry skin. This includes the nasal region that could be damaged. The other uses are the treatment of

- Diarrhea in daytime

- Nausea

Vertigo when standing

Herpes - Herpes

- Skin ulcers

Thuja Occidentalis

It is derived from the Arbor Vitae bush, thuja occidentalis is utilized to treat a variety of ailments . It is frequently a component of any homeopathic practitioner's initial aid kit. It has been in use for long periods of time, with the earliest usages being attributed to people of the Native Americans who used the plant to treat fevers and headaches, and coughs. Since then the variety of uses has increased with the advancement of studies and research:

- Cauliflower warts

Menstrual disorders that cause irregular flow

- Gonorrhea

- Sinusitis

- Chronic respiratory conditions

Aloe Socotrina

This remedy is made from the juices of the plant aloe vera. If taken internally, aloe sctorina can be used to treat diarrhea and colic. In older people it is taken to treat incontinence. In addition to these issues it can also be utilized to treat a variety of other ailments:

Prostate enlargement

- Weakness

- Tiredness

- Winter coughs

- Constipation

Gastritis

Chapter 4: Homeopathy And Nutrition

Homeopathy is definitely a feasible treatment option for a variety of ailments however, it's not a magic cure. It is not possible to take a pill or drink a concoction and be able to feel miraculously well. there are other aspects anyone who relies on Homeopathy should be able to do to ensure the effectiveness of the treatment plan. It is the same for Western medicines too. The patient must be on the right nutrition to achieve positive effects from any homeopathic treatment.

It's not only about eating healthy, it's also about selecting the best foods to eat. It is crucial that a healthy diet be followed in conjunction with any homeopathic treatment. Selecting organic meats, fruits and vegetables, or even cultivating your own is one method of achieving this. While supplements aren't always required but there are instances when they are required in order to make a person healthier enough to experience positive effects from the homeopathic treatments.

A diet that is rich in green leafy vegetables will always be an excellent thing. There are tons of nutrients in almost every fruit or vegetable that can help one feel better. Of sure there are some foods which are more nutritious than other ones. They are frequently called superfoods. Brightly colored vegetables can be very beneficial. It is best to eat organic meat and so is fish caught that are caught in the wild. Anyone who is eating an wholesome, balanced diet packed with nutritious foods won't need to supplement their diet. A lot of people are unaware that for a mineral or vitamin to perform at its best, it needs the support of another. That's why doctors constantly insist on healthy, balanced diets that include various foodsthat each contain each with a specific ingredient.

In the event that your food regimen is deficient of essential nutrients, using Spirulina could help compensate some of the nutrients you're likely to be lacking. This supplement is beneficial and has the essential nutrients required to improve the immune system and fighting cancer and allergies. Even though it's rich with protein it shouldn't be thought of as a substitute for protein. Instead, it's more of an enhancement to the already healthy diet.

When possible, it's recommended to eat fresh fruit and veggies. Processing or cooking for freezing or canning can cause a loss of nutrients. If we speak of having healthy food it's because we are trying to ensure that our body has adequate levels of the essential vitamins required for normal functioning.

The benefits of homeopathy

Many people steer clear of Homeopathic treatments due to ignorance of all the health benefits that it may offer and the role a Homeopathic remedy plays in the overall state of our health is not known.

Here are some of the benefits of Homeopathy:

It is a tool that can be used by almost everyone.

Children, pregnant women as well as the elderly could be benefited by this holistic treatment. Since the majority of the drugs used are dilute or are completely natural and suitable for all to use. But, to ensure that you are sure, it's usually recommended to speak with your Naturopath in order to determine whether Homeopathy is suitable for you.

When contrasted with other therapies which are employed by traditional medicine, Homeopathic treatments aren't causing structural harm to the body. They instead serve as a stimulant that helps to boost our body's inherent healing capabilities. They don't cause any chemical reactions that are not intended for the body, making them a reliable and safe element of every treatment regimen.

Do not interact with other medicines or treatments.

It is important to note that the Homeopathic treatments are weak and are in such small amounts that they are not likely to react with other medicines or treatments. Thus, you can utilize Homeopathic remedies along with other therapies.

Dosing the right amount is safe and don't cause health risks.

If you are given the wrong dose of a certain Homeopathic remedy It will not create an health risk or trigger any adverse reactions. The reason for this is that the dosages are low enough that they lack the power to harm the body.

Risk of side effects reduced.

In general, patients do not experience any adverse side effects at all. There have been instances where patients have experienced minor adverse reactions to specific treatments. These side effects tend to be temporary and typically manifest as worsened symptoms. When the symptoms are gone, patients generally will notice improvement in the symptoms and improved overall health.

This can be used in either long- or short-term needs.

Homeopathic remedies can be utilized for chronic as well as acute illnesses. Thus, those who suffer from both chronic and short-term problems can benefit from these remedies.

Treats all of the person.

Instead of just treating only the signs, whole patient is cared for. This means that the patient is evaluated and their overall health and well-being taken into account. This is not just an individual body part that gets looked after, but also the mental and emotional well-being of the patient also.

It is usually inexpensive and cost efficient.

The homeopathic remedies the doctor prescribes are typically less costly than the majority of traditional medications as well as other holistic treatments for healing including Ayurvedic treatments. The remedies that are Homeopathic can be stored for quite a long time, so there is no need to worry about it being wasted and is therefore cost-effective also. Additionally, the evaluation procedure in Homeopathy is much less expensive because the practitioner is not required to use a range of diagnostic tests in the exam.

It is non-invasive.

It doesn't require surgery or procedures that are invasive. So, you don't need to worry about any negative reactions or side effects which can result from anesthesia or the procedure itself. Additionally, there are no time frames for recovery.

Homeopathic remedies can be effective.

The advantages of Homeopathic remedies can be felt very quickly after treatment has started and they are usually very effective. When a patient is provided with an appropriate dosage of the most suitable remedy The benefits of the treatment could last, with signs not returning.

Aids, rather than inhibits the immune system, rather than hinders it.

In contrast to other types of treatment, like the prescription of certain drugs in conventional medicine, Homeopathic remedies aid in boosting the immune system instead of suppressing it. For instance, if suffer from a fever, and you are taking prescription medications, your fever will be reduced. But, the reason for the cause of the fever is the body's way of trying to eliminate the toxins which will make you more healthy and healthier in a shorter time.

Treatments aren't habit-forming.

The homeopathic remedies prescribed aren't habit-forming. Thus, you won't have to worry about developing an addiction to these medicines. If you've noticed benefits from the remedy and that the side effects are gone, you'll typically be able to discontinue taking the remedy.

Finds the root of the problem Not only the symptoms.

Because Homeopathy is able to treat the root of the issue and removes any symptoms associated with the illness It is not uncommon to have recurring problems once you've completed the treatment.

Homeopathic remedies are simple and quick to use.

The majority of homeopathic remedies are provided in convenient forms like pills or tablets. They are easy and simple to use. They are also suitable for those who are working, since they can be taken with the solution with you and use it when it is suggested to do so.

Homeopathy Treatment Method

If you're confused about what exactly you should be expecting during the process of Homeopathic treatment, then take a few minutes to go through this article. We'll go over the basic aspects of Homeopathic treatment plans and will also outline some of the aspects you need to remember during your Homeopathic treatment.

Looking for a certified expert...

When looking for the perfect homeopathic physician There are some aspects to take into consideration like the doctor's expertise and training. Also, make sure that they can manage your specific health problem and also provide the treatment options that you're thinking about. For instance, if you are suffering from migraines that persist for a long time it is recommended to find a doctor who is specialized in chronic headaches or pain and can provide you with the best treatment plan specific to your kind of migraine. This will ensure that you receive the maximum benefit from your treatment , and also the doctor you choose is the best fit to your particular health requirements.

Making preparations for the first appointment and the Diagnosis Procedure...

When you make an appointment with your homeopathic physician to the first time arrive at least a few minutes earlier to complete the paperwork required. Also, you should write an inventory of your symptoms prior to your appointment, so that you'll be able to include all of them when your doctor asks about your health issues currently. When you visit your doctor they will ask you about your overall health status including your physical, emotional and mental health. The doctor may also ask you to provide a health history and take a physical examination. Some health care professionals will require you to take the blood test or submit the urine sample to have a better understanding of your health. They'll then provide you with the prescription for a Homeopathic remedy based on all the data gathered.

It is also important to keep in mind that in Homeopathy patients are an integral element of the process of treatment. You should take an active part in your care because the process of healing is heavily dependent on your body's ability to self-heal. The treatment you'll be offered is just meant to activate your body's immune system. So, it is important to be truthful and open when describing the symptoms you are experiencing to your health care physician and inform them of any concerns that you may have. Make sure you inform them of the specific issue that hinders you from living more fulfilled life. For instance, even when you see a doctor for stomach pain make sure you mention any mental or emotional issues you are having. Although these issues might not be relevant but they could play a part in the development of your illness.

How are Remedies administered...

Homeopathic remedies can be given in various ways. The method used to administer them will depend on the preference of the patient as will the components that were used to make the remedy. The primary forms that remedies are offered comprise gels, creams tablets, pellets and liquids.

Tablet. This kind of treatment is usually soft and is made up of the sugar of milk (lactose). The remedy is perfect for infants and young children as it is more easy for them to swallow. It also dissolves quickly.

Creams/Gels. These treatments are usually less potent and aren't intended to be consumed. They are instead designed to be applied directly (on your skin) to treat symptoms that are external.

Liquids. These kinds of remedies are intended to be consumed orally and are extremely powerful. It is recommended to take a minimum of one hour before brushing your teeth and then 30 minutes before you consume food following the oral versions of remedies.

Pellets. This remedy is taken orally and is typically applied to the tongues of patients. Pellets may be crushed, or dissolve in water.

A Follow-up...

Once you have started receiving treatment After receiving treatment, you are asked for follow-up appointments. They are typically scheduled between a month and 2 months apart contingent on what your healthcare provider suggests. The follow-up visits provide the doctor with a chance to assess how the treatment is working and also to determine if a new treatment or a higher dosage should be prescribed. Although some patients might find that one remedy works and can eliminate the symptoms completely, other patients may find that a long treatment is required. There are many benefits to adhering to the treatment once the right treatment is discovered, such as an improvement or complete elimination of symptoms, increased levels of energy, improved well-being and better sleeping.

What to Do to...

If you are using Homeopathic remedies, you should be aware of certain substances to avoid. These are known in the field of "antidotes" of the remedies. They essentially counteract the beneficial effect of the cure, or make them ineffective. Although you may begin using the remedy after it has been treated with an antidote medication, the treatment procedure is usually more challenging and time-consuming. Thus, you must stay away from the following ingredients:

Coffee or extremely caffeinated drinks.

Camphor-containing substances such as essential oils of eucalyptus.

The procedure of dental work must also be avoided. This is due to the use of anesthetics and drilling frequently used in these procedures can hamper your recovery when the patient is taking Homeopathic treatments.

High levels of stress. This is because stress-inducing events, like an illness or death can impede the effects of the treatment.

Things to be aware of...

There are many things to bear in mind when you are considering homeopathic remedies. First of all, you shouldn't utilize Homeopathy as a substitute for conventional medical care or avoid visiting a physician in the event of a major health problem. If you're considering trying a remedy, bring it along to the next appointment with your doctor to learn the doctor's opinion on the remedy and make sure it is suitable for you and your health requirements. Your doctor can also to inform you if other remedies are better suited for your medical condition.

When you take the Homeopathic remedy, you must be sure to adhere to the dosage guidelines carefully. In addition despite the fact that Homeopathy can be used by all however, if you're nursing or pregnant, or plan to treat children with the remedy, you must consult with your physician prior to doing it. Also, you must inform all health care professionals who are part of your treatment plan the different types of therapy that you're employing. This gives them an opportunity to look at how your general health is affected and your treatment plan of action, which means they can make better choices.

Wellness Treatments with complimentary Holistic Complimentary

As an holistic health professional I thought it would be beneficial to dedicate a part of this manual to the treatments that are a good complement to Homeopathy. There are a myriad of remedies for healing using nature that will help you maximize the benefits of the Homeopathic treatments, since they can help enhance the connection between the mind and body, and allow your body to start healing itself. I strongly suggest you look into the following natural remedies while you're preparing your treatment plan, since each one has the potential to increase the efficacy of Homeopathy.

Massage Therapy

I am (and always will continue to be) an avid advocate of massage therapy. Massage is one of the ways that massage therapy was my first introduction to the field of holistic health. It will always be among my top choices of the best complementary therapies therefore, I could be biased when I claim that massage is among the best methods to relax or stress relief as well as general improvement in health. But, it can be even more effective alongside Homeopathy.

There are several massage techniques to think about that range in range from Swedish up to Shiatsu. Each comes with its own advantages. To give you a clear idea of what each kind can provide this is a quick overview of the most well-known types of massages:

Swedish.

Swedish massage is the first thing that is the first thing people's mind when they think of massages. It usually involves slow movements that aid in stretching muscles and ease any tension that might have built up in the muscles. It also helps to ease tension in the body and mind. When you go to the typical Swedish massage it is suggested that you undress and drape yourself so you don't get exposed to any part. The therapist will apply an oil, cream or lotion to give enough glide while performing the techniques of massage.

Swedish massage consists of four specific techniques: effleurage friction, tapotement, and effleurage. Effleurage is characterized by long strokes and petrissage involves kneading the muscle and tissue. Friction improves circulation and helps to relax the muscles and tapotement utilizes quick precise hitting strokes to help tone the muscle. This kind of massage is perfect for people who are experiencing mental or physical stress. It is also able to increase the efficacy of homeopathic remedies designed to heal the body and mind.

Shiatsu.

Shiatsu was developed in Japan and is an extremely sought-after types of massages across the globe today. The client is completely covered during a shiatsu massage practice, and the therapist uses finger pressure instead of moving in a fluid manner. Shiatsu massage relies on the concept that we all have energy meridians that flow through the body. An Shiatsu massage therapist presses and hold certain meridians along these meridians in order in order to restore equilibrium and remove any obstructions that could hinder the flow of energy.

Hot Stone.

Hot stone massages generally include Swedish massage techniques that are utilized in conjunction with hot stones. The stones are typically warmed prior to the beginning of the session, and the practitioner applies them to different areas of the body. Some practitioners will simply put the stones on certain areas in the human body for instance, around your spine. They employ their hands to carry out the massage. Others may prefer using stones that are hot for massage of the client. The hot stone massage may assist in relieving muscle pain and improve circulation.

Deep Tissue.

Massages that are deep in the tissue can be utilized by those who would prefer a more intense pressure during their massage, or people who suffer from knots that are larger. This kind of massage permits the practitioner to get deeper into the tissues and muscles that can help remove knots and tight muscles. Certain techniques employed during a deep tissue massage could involve massaging the muscle within the muscle itself, using the form of a cross-fiber movement. This method helps release tension stored within the muscle tissue that can offer almost instant relief to the patient.

The main reason massage is a good option for people who are using Homeopathic remedies is the fact that it aids to improve the immune system, as well as helps to relax the body and mind. This allows remedies to work to work their "magic," given that they will not have to contend with the stressors that normally hinder healing, because massage helps you relax and decrease stress levels.

Meditation

Some people might not see this as a holistic method in and of itself, because it doesn't require assistance from a qualified expert to enjoy the benefits that meditation can bring (as this is more of a self-help method). But, I see that as an extremely effective holistic treatments for healing. If you give it a bit of consideration, you will are able to see Homeopathy is about letting your body heal itself by activating your body's healing processes. Meditation, in its essence is a type of relaxation that can allow you to let your body relax and receive the time, attention, and time it requires to take care of itself. This is why it's the ideal complement to natural remedies.

There isn't a specific type of meditation you have to apply to your treatment there isn't a guidelines regarding how to do it to reap the greatest benefits. It is a completely personal experience that requires you to modify. It could be that being in your space for a few minutes each day brings you enormous satisfaction, or you may realize that you will benefit the most from a lengthy practice that you dedicate an hour every day. The type of meditation you select to practice and how often you go through it, is a totally individual choice. Below I've given you some tips to help you meditate, so that you'll get an idea of how to begin the practice of meditation that is your own.

Learn the art of mindful breathing.

Focusing and breathing may appear as if they come naturally to you. But, you might discover it to be difficult to concentrate upon your breath and to concentrate on the stream of thoughts. These are two fundamental elements of meditation since they permit you to spend time in a state of relaxation and clear your mind and observe your breathing patterns and also the thoughts that might hinder your healing process.

Find time to practice meditation.

If you're just beginning to meditate begin by taking some time your day to dedicate to meditation. It's essential to take space for yourself so that you can reflect on your morning and refresh your thoughts. If you're lucky enough to have the time you can sit in a calm location and take a deep breath in , then exhale slowly. It will be apparent that, initially the breaths you take are quick and thin. This is usually due to the stress that you're experiencing, possibly because most of us live fast-paced lives. Take a moment to inhale until you feel your lungs are completely expanded and then slowly let breathe out.

Get rid of worry and negative thoughts.

While you make efforts to concentrate upon your breath, be sure that your mind is free of stress or negativity. Let go of any worries that you've accumulated to let the mind unwind completely. It might be difficult to simply let go of your thoughts and let it go, so it's better to imagine that you're in a serene, quiet place that is serene and serene (this is sometimes referred to in the field of visualization).

Aromatherapy

If you encounter the term "aromatherapy," they may immediately think it's just a scent-infused candle or bubble bath can be used to unwind and relax after an exhausting day. But, it goes beyond that, and offers numerous advantages, from stress relief to pain relief for chronic conditions. In actual fact it has been utilized throughout the world over the centuries, with people from all over the world making use of it to supply them with the benefits of essential oils that are all-natural. Some oils also have the capability of relieving illnesses and improve overall health.

While oils that are utilized in room sprays or diffusers are often confused with Aromatherapy oils, real aromatherapy oils are completely different ingredients. Essential oils for aromatherapy are the pure oils obtained directly from the source and usually are not diluted. Instead of being used as fragrances the oils are made for their benefits both mentally and physically.

To benefit from the oils, you need to know the benefits of each one and also the best way to be used. For instance, if need an instant boost of energy, the essential oils of citrus such as lemon or orange is a good choice. It is also helpful to mix these oils with creams for massage during massage therapy or inhaling the aroma while receiving other holistic therapies.

Here are some of the benefits which are typically linked to aromatherapy:

- It increases blood flow and allows the elimination of toxins of the body. This will help to strengthen the immune system. This will allow Homeopathic remedies be more effective and efficient.

It is a good antibacterial agent. This can allow you stay away from the flu and cold as well as enhance your overall well-being.

It boosts energy levels and allows you to concentrate on the job that is at hand. It also improves stamina and decreases fatigue.

Relaxes the physique and mental state, which allows you to increase your enjoyment of living.

One of the most appealing aspects with aromatherapy is it can incorporate it easily into your everyday routine. Do you want to burn candles with essential oils when you're feeling stressed or put a few on your bed prior to getting ready to sleep in order to have a more peaceful sleep? It is also possible to consult your holistic health professional to make use of essential oils during your treatments to increase the effects of these treatments as well.

Yoga

Yoga has been practiced for a long time, and is frequently utilized to improve the quality of life and reduce stress. There are many different types of yoga you can select from, however each one has one feature in the same: they bring your mind and body together and assist you in achieving an overall balance and also improve your health. Yoga is a popular choice for many to ease stress levels, improve your mood and outlook, and boost your mental clarity.

The best method to get the most benefits of yoga practice is to discover the right type of yoga that suits you and your specific needs.

Here's a short overview of some styles of yoga that are widely used in the present:

Hatha.

The practice of yoga as it is known today was developed around the time of the 15th century. It is perfect for people who are just beginning because of its focus on the most basic poses as well as relaxation methods. It can help relieve stress as well as improve your physical health and improve your breathing habits. Hatha is also able to enhance the effectiveness of homeopathic remedies (as all types of yoga can do) by enhancing your body-mind connection, and enhancing your overall relaxation.

Vinyasa.

This form of yoga is focused on synchronizing your breathing and your movements. Vinyasa is a set of 12 poses known as the'sun salutation in which each of your movements is linked to breathing. It aids in building muscles, increase endurance, increase flexibility and decrease the risk of developing some serious diseases like hypertension and heart disease.

Bikram.

It is among the most difficult, considering the fact that it's performed in rooms where temperatures can vary from 95 to 100 degrees F. This is why it's frequently referred to as hot yoga. It involves the practice of 26 poses, all of which is specifically designed to stretch the muscles and eliminate toxins that naturally build up in the body. It is ideal for people who are trying to shed weight and seeking a method to detoxify their body's systems.

Acupuncture

Acupuncture has been utilized throughout the ages as a means to relieve pain and as a natural treatment particularly throughout the Eastern World. Many thousands of years ago practitioners from all over China used acupuncture to prolong life and cure common diseases. In a typical acupuncture session practitioners insert tiny, sterilized needles in specific points located throughout the body. These points are chosen with care because each one corresponds to a specific organ, system or.

There are two different ways of thinking as it relates to the way acupuncture operates. There are a variety of Western doctors believe needles stimulate nerves in addition to your muscles and tissues. However traditional Chinese medical practitioners believe that acupuncture can help regulate the flow of energy (energy meridians) throughout your body. Acupuncturists believe that putting needles in precisely chosen areas will help restore balance to the movement of energy. People who suffer from various diseases, like back pain and asthma might experience regular acupuncture sessions as beneficial, and so will those taking homeopathic treatments.

Reiki

Reiki is also a firm believer in the notion that, you are given the chance, your body is able to recover itself. In actual fact, Reiki practitioners believe that the body's energy could be an energy source for healing. Reiki was developed in Japan which is where it was first developed in 1922. It has been used to decrease tension and ease pain since then, across many regions of the world. In a typical session an Reiki practitioner applies their fingers or hands directly over or on the body of the patient using massaging movements to release energy or increase an energy flow to treat.

The patient is usually requested to lie down or to be moved into a comfortable position (if they're unable to lay down). The Reiki treatment is performed completely covered, which means it's not necessary to remove your clothes during a session. Instead of focusing solely on the problem area the practitioner will typically perform a series of hand movements or techniques for positioning throughout the body. This is because Reiki addresses the entire person and not only the symptoms (much as Homeopathy is similar to Homeopathy).

Reiki is an excellent supplement to Homeopathic remedies as it is able to help those suffering with acute or chronic pain and emotional and mental issues. The less complicated injuries might just require a couple of sessions, whereas more severe illnesses may require regular Reiki sessions.

Reflexology

Reflexology is ideal for those looking for an effective method to ease chronic pain and also for patients suffering from an acute issue. The practitioners of reflexology apply pressure on certain points on the patients' feet, hands or the ear. The premise behind reflexology is that every of these points is related to a specific region in the body. Or the organs of the body. By pressing these important points, the specific area that is part of your human body (or some of its main systems) which is associated with it will be relieved or assisted by the treatment.

Reflexology isn't typically employed to diagnose or treat a specific problem. However, it is employed as a treatment complement. It is beneficial to add it to a treatment program which includes homeopathic remedies to further assist the patient. People suffering from anxiety, asthma or chronic pain kidney problems can benefit from the reflexology treatment and patients suffering from certain heart issues.

Sound therapy

Sound therapy is unique because it's one of the only therapies which you are likely to engage in every day. Sound therapy could be that is as easy as listening to a relaxing classic piece in the comfort of your home space, or as complex as visiting an expert sound therapy. In a sound therapy session you might experience a particular genre of music or the therapist may make more intriguing sounds like the drum and chant. In reality the majority of sound therapy practitioners use a range of auditory stimuli in order to get the desired results. For instance, old singing bowls are employed to help calm the mind and ease anxiety.

The objective of the sound therapy session is to boost the quality of life and lessen stress. But, it is also a method to reduce a range of common conditions, including migraines and back pain. To determine whether sound therapy is suitable for you, then it is possible to start by having an audiotherapy session at home. Sit in a calm space and put on some music that is relaxing (at the lowest volume). Simply focus on the music and attempt to let go of all negative thoughts.

Color Therapy

Even though we might not be conscious of it, colors play an essential part in our lives. Certain colors may aid us in attaining specific effects in our bodies, minds as well as emotionally. For instance, the yellow color can boost our energy levels and the color red can inspire imagination. The mere act of wearing a certain colour or changing the color of your bedding will significantly affect your mood. Therapists also specialize in a method called"chromotherapy. In chromotherapy, patients are treated with a variety of shades of light, in order to improve their overall well-being and perspective on living.

The session with color therapy will usually take place in a dark room. The therapist then applies light to different parts within the human body. The devices that are typically employed are colored slides and essences placed on the skin as well as lamps that emit different colors of light, and low-level laser therapy. The colors the therapist chooses to use are based on the mood or health issue or condition of the person.

You could even perform an exercise in color therapy at your home. Just change the paint on your walls or take a look at pictures that show hues that can create the desired effects. This will help you change your perception , and also increase the effectiveness of your homeopathic remedies.

Chapter 5: The Debunking Of Popular Myths

About Homeopathy

There are many myths you could encounter in your research on Homeopathy. Actually some of these myths have been all over the place for so long they've become the norm for some (especially people who're skeptical regarding holistic health and Homeopathy or opponents on Homeopathic cures). So, I thought I'd use this time to dispel the most popular myths and expose the truth behind them.

It refers to "magic" and is employed to treat anything.

It's one of the most well-known myths I've encountered on the web in recent times. The majority of the time, this myth is circulated by less than trustworthy sites selling products that claim their products are designed to "cure whatever ails you." The issue with these websites is that they often than not fail to please their clients and customers, not to mention their fact that they make Homeopathy an unpopular name. As there isn't a magic potion that can bring youth (at the very least, so that I can tell) There isn't a magic potion that will solve everything. There are certain illnesses or conditions which require surgery or other extreme medical procedures.

While Homeopathic remedies are effective in capability to treat different diseases and boost the overall health of your body, with out the possibility of side consequences, there are instances where medical attention is required. For instance, if someone is diagnosed with a life-threatening condition, such as an illness that is a tumor or a form of cancer, it typically calls for more extensive medical treatments which are not within the scope of Homeopathic medical treatment.

Homeopathy is only used to treat chronic conditions.

Another myth I've heard a lot of times in relation to the notion that Homeopathy is only used to treat chronic, long-term ailments but not for conditions who require immediate care (such as headaches or diarrhea). This isn't the reality; in reality, there are numerous Homeopathic remedies designed to be used only for acute conditions. Homeopathy can be quick-acting and efficient in treating illness such as colds and flu, so that they can provide instant relief from symptoms.

The problem that plagues the majority of sufferers is the fact that many do not seek the assistance of a homeopathic physician until their chronic condition becomes chronic. This is a contributing factor to the myth. But, when patients let acute issues to develop into chronic health problems it is possible that their conditions be more difficult to be treated. Additionally, many patients are reluctant to seek Homeopathy after all other treatments have been unsuccessful (which could be another cause people are misled into thinking that Homeopathy is only suitable for people suffering with chronic ailments). If the patients had sought out Homeopathic treatment before they started it could have stopped their condition from developing into chronic.

The main point is this: Homeopathic remedies are effective in treating both chronic and acute ailments.

Homeopathic remedies are, most typically, nothing more than placebos.

This particular story is one I've heard for a long time. It's also the one that's the most concerning to me. This is because it causes me to wonder what percentage of people are avoiding turning to Homeopathic treatment because they believe it's just "sugar pill" and "magic serums" that are sold from "snake oil sellers."

When I first started with my practice (which included Aromatherapy and massage at that time) I had a patient that I visited regularly. She was always scheduled to see me , and she firmly believed in the healing process that was natural. She was visiting massage therapists for a long time and was convinced that aromatherapy and massage therapy and many other holistic treatments were essential to an improvement in the level of living. But despite the fact that the client was so engrossed in the healing philosophy of natural healing however, she was unable to seek help from an Homeopathic physician.

I also spent the time to inform that she could reap the rewards it might bring and then went over the different remedies I suggested.

97

But she was stubborn and was unwilling to try it until she started experiencing severe headaches. After two weeks of continuous and debilitating headaches she made an appointment for an emergency with me. Although I was aware that she had tight muscles in her trapezius and scalene which could cause headaches, I was not sufficient to offer her immediate relief for her severe headache. So, I suggested she visit one of my friends who was the Homeopathic doctor who had introduced me to Homeopathy several years prior when she finally accepted.

The following week, she went to see me again , and was completely free of headaches. As soon as I started taking a look at me, it was easy to see she was happy and healthier. The colour returned to her cheeks and it was as if an enormous weight was removed from her shoulders. She spoke to me about her visit to the homeopathic doctor as well as the remedy she was given. She'd tried various over-the counter headache medicines and other treatments that are holistic like acupuncture, however, all that brought her immediate relief and lasting relief is the treatment. She thanked me for more than I can remember for and referred her to my friend. She also acknowledged that she ought to have tried Homeopathy several years ago.

Then I finally understood why she was so opposed to the concept of Homeopathy. She then told me that she was persuaded that Homeopathy was just a bunch of "hogwash" which offered its most unlucky clients placebos (that cost a lot). At some point she'd been told that Homeopathy is ineffective which had kept her from trying it. There are thousands of others just like her, who've been told Homeopathy is ineffective and has nothing to offer other than false claims as well as "snake oils."

Another reason for me to write this book. The truth is that homeopathy can, in fact can treat a variety of diseases, if people would stop believing in the myths disseminated and open their mind to the options for treatment.

Patients taking Homeopathic remedies must adhere to extremely strict diets.

Although there are certain food items and substances to be avoided, for instance caffeine, you don't have to adhere to any specific diet when using Homeopathic remedies. The reason that certain items are classified as "off boundaries" is because they interfere to enhance the effect of certain remedies. For instance, some drugs might lose their potency if you consume alcohol or smoking while taking them.

As I mentioned in the previous chapter, even though it is true it isn't a requirement to adhere to diet limitations, it's still recommended to follow an optimum diet when you're doing Homeopathic cures (and even after you've been treated or any other remedy for that matter). This will allow you to increase your overall well-being and boost your overall health to strengthen your body and mind.

There is no scientific evidence for Homeopathic remedies.

This is not the reality. When it comes to the creation of new Homeopathic remedies are being developed in the first place, they have to go through a scientific "proving" procedure, in it is administered to test group comprising at least 50 people. The volunteers are all healthy and are instructed to use the remedy for a specified trial period of time until they show symptoms. The participants must document their symptoms as precisely as they can, and submit their findings which are then entered into the database. In most cases, participants are provided with tests that fall within the 30C range of potency.

Participants must meet certain requirements and follow specific rules throughout the trial. They must be healthy prior to starting the trial and they shouldn't talk to any other participants regarding their ailments. When this trial, every one the symptoms experienced by the majority of participants are included in those listed as symptoms that are associated with the remedy. These symptoms are included in the Materia the Medicas of Homeopathic remedies along with the Homeopathic Repertory that is best described as an Encyclopedia of Homeopathic symptoms.

The Homeopathic Materia Medica and the Homeopathic Repertory contain a huge amount of information. In fact they are so extensive that the Homeopathic Repertory is so large that it's split into sections, which include (in order) Vertigo, Mind, Head Eye, Vision Ear, Hearing Nose Face, Mouth Teeth

Throat External Throat Stomach, Abdomen Rectum Bladder, Stool Prostate Gland Urethra, Urine, Male Female, Larynx Respiration, Cough, Expectoration Chest, Back Sleep, Dreams, Extremities Chill, Fever generals, skin, sweat.

The Homeopathic Repertories listed remedies are listed alongside the related symptoms (which are all written in an abbreviated format). In these publications there is a listing of every emotion human being experiences, every physical condition, as well as every mental state. Each possible symptom is described in order to be identified and the remedy that will be utilized as a remedy can be recommended by the doctor to treat the person. This is the thing that makes Homeopathy so fascinating It's not only about the disease as such, but also the symptoms, and even the mental state that could be causing the illness.

A variety of substances have been examined, including minerals and metals that are listed on the periodic table , to more extreme elements like snake venom (there are over 4,500 Homeopathic cures that are identified and documented). There have been even accidental poisonings that were added to the extensive database of symptoms that could be triggered, like those experienced by those who have been in contact with arsenic. This database of symptoms permits doctors to identify which treatment will ease a specific group of symptoms. For instance the patient seeks help from a homeopathic physician due to diarrhea and vomiting that have resulted from food poisoning, the doctor might suggest Arsenicum to help eliminate the symptoms.

Homeopathic remedies aren't as effective as prescription medications.

The final myth I'd like to debunk is the belief that homeopathic remedies aren't as efficient as prescription drugs or that they're ineffective. The truth is that Homeopathy assists in healing by stimulating and boosting the body's body's immune system as well as the healing. Every person is able to recover if they are provided with the proper signal. In many instances all you require is a trigger to trigger your healing chain reaction inside your body and your mind.

In contrast to traditional medical approaches, Homeopathy focuses on curing the root cause of the issue instead of just dealing with the symptoms. Therefore, people who use Homeopathic treatments often notice that they are able to enjoy long-lasting relief from their condition and can achieve this without worrying about any negative side effects that conventional prescription medications can trigger. In essence, homeopathic remedies provide you with the power to heal regardless of whether you suffer from chronic or acute illness.

Homeopathy FAQ

What makes Homeopathy different in comparison to Traditional Medicine?

There are several ways Homeopathy differentiates itself from other forms of medical. For one, when using Homeopathic remedies patients are considered to be an individual instead of merely the manifestation of symptoms. This means that the patient's total wellbeing is considered to be taken care of in addition to their physical health. Furthermore, every treatment plan and treatment is customized for the individual so that they can eliminate any symptoms as well as the root of their issue. Instead of receiving an medication which is administered to everyone suffering from the specific ailment and the patient is provided an individual treatment plan in which the dosage's effectiveness is individualized for his or her.

Here's an illustration of how a treatment plan could differ between traditional and homeopaths doctors:

A patient is suffering from frequent and severe headaches that are affecting his ability to perform on a daily basis. He decides to seek the assistance of a doctor when the pain becomes for him to handle.

What would occur if he relied on traditional medicine? The doctor may ask how often he's experiencing headaches and examine the medical records of his patient to look up his past. The doctor will then issue a prescription for a drug that is prescribed to all patients suffering frequently from headaches.

What would happen if he was to rely on Homeopathic treatment? Patients would likely be asked questions about his medical history before receiving an exam. The doctor would seek out more information about the patient's psychological healthand inquire about the specifics related to the headache. In particular, the doctor might need to know the exact time the headaches begin, as well as whether the patient is suffering from other symptoms, such as fever or nausea. The physician would then provide the patient an appropriate prescription that comes with a specific dosage and ingredients that match the patient's needs.

What are the symptoms that are evaluated in an Homeopathy appointment?

Instead of just looking for information on an individual symptom you are worried about or a specific symptom, a Homeopathic practitioner is likely to know the full extent of any and all signs you've observed. Although it is possible to believe that all the symptoms are not related, in reality you'll find that they may be connected to a common reason. There are many patients who experience frequent symptoms that change for example, headaches that only affect the sufferer when they're in the sunlight for too long or discomforts and aches that occur not frequent, but they are a nuisance. When you see a practitioner of Homeopathy be sure to mention all of these issues.

Here are a few of the signs that a doctor might want to be aware about:

The most obvious symptom which is often the reason you came in for the first time.

Things or events that cause your symptoms to get worse or better.

In what areas of your body feel these symptoms.

The time when the symptoms first began and what could have led to the initial occurrence of the symptoms.

Your current state of mind.

The texture and color the stool. Also, how often do you are able to bowel during the day.

If you're asleep well or awake frequently throughout the night.

What things are you sensitive to, for example, light, cold, or others' comments?

If you're having difficulties in any aspect or aspect of life. For example, are you struggling with relationships or sexual issues. ?

What are the most common applications of homeopathic treatment?

There are three major reasons to use Homeopathy. They are commonly described as "levels" in the treatment. You may pay a visit to an Homeopath in any one of the following reasons:

First Aid. It is recommended to seek the advice from an Homeopathic specialist for health issues that are common to all including minor burns, bruises skin irritations, or injuries. It is also possible to visit one in case you're suffering from an allergic reaction, such as insect bites or diaper rash or exposure to poisonous plants.

Acute homeopathy (short word). Acute health conditions can be described as issues which could disappear by themselves provided they're given enough time. They can be short-term or temporary problems like common colds and flu. If you decide to seek help from a Homeopath or a Homeopath, then you'll be able to accelerate the recovery of these illnesses and discover more about why you could be suffering from them in the first instance. For instance, if you see a practitioner of homeopathy to treat an illness like cough, he/ they can determine the reason you're coughing and attempt to pinpoint the source of the problem.

Constitutional Homeopathy (long term). This type of permanent Homeopathy is intended to treat the entire person through the creation of a constitutional Homeopathy treatment program. Your present symptoms are evaluated along with your experiences previously. This type of holistic treatment can address chronic pain issues and also boost your immune system to ensure that you don't experience the same symptoms in the future.

How can the small dosages of medication be efficacious?

Despite the fact the doses of medicine you'll be given during the course of your homeopathic treatment are low however, they're extremely efficient. The reason for this is that the medicines are subject to a specific procedure of preparation (which was explained in the earlier book). This process is referred to as "potentization" and can make even small amounts of your medication very potent. The remedies aid your body recover itself by encouraging it to fight against what is causing the symptoms you're experiencing.

How can I get included in how I can be involved in Homeopathic Treatment Plan?

Every patient who chooses to use homeopathic remedies must be actively active in their self-healing process. The patient should be honest in answering the questions the doctor asks to the highest of their abilities. This will ensure that the patient receives the best high-quality care since the physician will have a complete and precise picture of all the signs and symptoms in the treatment, not only the most obvious. Also, monitor the changes that take place in the course of the treatments you are taking, and inform your healthcare provider of the changes. This will help the physician to make any necessary changes to your treatment.

It is also important to ensure that you do not use any substances that be used like an "antidote" to the remedy. Antidotes may impede the benefits the remedy is providing and can render it completely ineffective. Camphor, caffeine products and dental work blankets and nicotine, mentholated items medications, certain prescribed medication, x-rays, as well as excessive levels of stress are all to be avoided when you're using a Homeopathic remedy.

Are Homeopathy protected by health insurance?

In general, Homeopathic treatments are not covered by health insurance companies. It is recommended you speak with your health insurance provider to find out if your particular treatments are covered. If you have to pay for it out on your own, you'll be relieved to know that Homeopathy is generally less expensive than other types of treatment. It is due to the fact that it offers the option of healing without costly medication or surgical procedures that require time to recover (and delayed work). A lot of patients find that their symptoms don't come back after taking Homeopathic remedies, which implies that they are not required to purchase additional medication or treatments later on for the specific ailment.

What are the things I must keep in mind while using my homeopathic remedies?

If you are administering the Homeopathic treatments, it might be helpful to have these guidelines in your pocket:

The medications that come in tablet form must be placed on the tongue, and then allowed to dissolve. If you're taking medication which are in the form of drops then you must administer them by using a small amount of water (approximately half one cup).

Your mouth must be clean after you take the remedy. This can be accomplished by washing it by drinking water prior to taking the remedy.

Beware of drinking, eating or smoking immediately following the time you have taken your medication, and prior to giving it.

Make sure to handle the remedy the least amount you can in order to prevent contamination.

If you're not comfortable with the way you administer your remedy inform your homeopathic doctor. He or she might be competent to prescribe the remedy in a different way.

How do I store my remedies from Homeopathy?

When you've received your Homeopathic treatment via the pharmacist, keep in mind the following storage guidelines:

If you're Homeopathic medication comes in tablets, they will be used for many years if it is stored correctly. They are composed of liquid and will be the same shelf life as alcohol as one of the primary liquid ingredients.

Keep the lid on the containers you use for remedy tight to ensure that they're well-protected.

If the solution is in a glass container, be sure to keep it out of the direct light.

Do not store your medicine in an area with many unpleasant smells, such as the kitchen pantry or bathroom.

There's no reason to keep your remedy within the fridge. In reality, they can be kept at the room temperature.

Don't place your homeopathic medication near electronic devices like your television or phone.

Chapter 6: Homeopathy's Principles

1.1 Why choose HOMEOPATHY?

If you go to your G.P. the reason why he might be writing a prescription on a pad while you are in his office is because you might have an idea of what he'll prescribe to you prior to the time he meets you. You've probably been able to inform the receptionist you, for instance, are suffering from influenza. By that label, it is clear that you have a cold that is shivering pain in your limbs, headache and more. These are all common symptoms of the illness we call influenza, so 90 percent of the doctor's work is done to diagnose. There is a chance that he'll observe an additional symptom that could result in him putting another label on whatever you're suffering from however, regardless of the method of determining the diagnosis after a label has been placed on a disease, that patient will receive the same medications as other patient with the same condition the doctor observed during the week. Sometimes it is just as easy to contact and have a prescription given to you 'on the board for you based solely according to your diagnosis.

Diagnostics is the primary element of Western Medicine, the largest portion of the money that is set aside for research is spent creating diagnostic tools like scanning devices, microscopes with electrons and so on. Of obviously, these are fantastic inventions that allow us to see the inner workings in the human body in greater depth, however the issues associated with these methods of diagnosis are numerous. While you focus on an small area of your body; patients as a person are likely to be omitted. Once the results in the diagnosis tests comes through and your medical condition is given an appropriate label, you are added to the list of patients who were given the same labeland will receive identical treatment.

When you go to the homeopath, you will notice that he'll take notes for a lengthy time taking notes and be able to ask questions. He's curious about the way you feel about things, and how you respond to your illness. He's not trying to find an identifiable condition, but rather is fascinated by how you with your illness is different from others. In essence, you are a unique individual and it is based upon the uniqueness of your personality, which is you and only you which he'll choose the right medicines to prescribe.

"Allopathy, Orthodox medical practice treating diseases with medications, etc. and whose effects on the body is in opposition to that of the disease different by homeopathy." The Chambers Twentieth Century Dictionary, examines a patient in order to determine if a disease is present and then give it a name . this process, it limits the uniqueness of the patient, thereby reducing the chance of identifying odd, unique and unusual symptoms. For illustration consider the case of an individual who, 14 years ago was identified with Multiple Sclerosis. The diagnosis was based due to the condition that from time period, around twice a year, she experienced an intense paralysis on one side that made walking difficult and lasted for between 3 and 4 days and were followed by headaches. followed by irritability. On every occasion, they occurred during the week before the start of her Menstrual Period and then stopped when the menstrual cycle began.

The woman has been identified as "Multiple Sclerosis for the past 14 years. This has affected her ability to receive life insurance as well as her auto insurance policy is packed. If medical professionals had asked her about these unusualities in relation to when and that the attacks began and related conditions, I wonder whether she would have been classified as 'M.S."?

The correct homeopathic treatment takes all of these elements into consideration and the result was that this woman is symptom-free for many years.

The homeopathic approach is to observe the patient and to identify the signs which define the uniqueness of the patient. It broadens the scope of the 'flu' that the doctor observes to encompass the completeness that the person has.

Disease, as we've been taught to believe, is a myth. it is not real. Let me clarify, it is not possible to catch cold, but we have been taught to believe that way, to think of that a disease is in the shadows, waiting to be discovered in the event that we are foolish enough to be caught in a cold. This kind of conditioning, even a part of our communication, can make it hard to change our ways of thinking.

When we say that"a person has" flu, we're ignoring the uniqueness of the individual. It's more accurate to say this person, due to stress, stress-related factors, surroundings and conditions that are unique to him only is causing an array of symptoms. These symptoms suggest it is an internal issue. If we look at these symptoms on their own without considering the other symptoms the set of symptoms are similar to the symptoms that are manifested by a different group of people's.

Although that's more precise and thorough description of the situation , it is infinitely more convenient to simply declare that 'He's got the flu' and so we just take the simplest route and continue to employ words that define our understanding of the world.

This system of telling a patient that he's 'got' or "caught" something comes with several interesting side consequences - it shifts any the responsibility for his condition from the patient and makes him believe that the disease once "caught" will be eliminated through the ingestion of substances in the body (chemicals or poisons, vitamins or special foods, for example.) The patient is also urged not to understand the rhythm and functioning of his body, to investigate his own habits or change his lifestyle.

It isn't quantifiable. it's not a 'thing that can be measured, but it is an indication of an individual's inability to adapt to changes emotionally, morally or psychologically. He is not in control of his own resource budget. The inner imbalance results in waves that hit the surface in the form of signs.

What are symptoms? As per the New Standard Dictionary by Funk and Wagnell"Symptoms" are "A symptoms. The thing that serves to demonstrate the existence of another thing an indication, token or sign."

What are we trying to say in this case? When someone is sick, it's because of an imbalance. The physical manifestations or effects we feel are just the body's normal responses to this internal problem. How do we manage these signs?

Illustrations can assist us in thinking about this issue.

In the year 1982 Britain had been at war with Argentina on the Falkland Islands. The inhabitants of those areas of the British Isles were made aware of events on the opposite side of the globe through broadcasts, T.V, radio and newspapers as in addition to those who returned from abroad and describing their personal experiences.

If we can compare the conflict and the build of it to an invisible internal disease, and the news of the war that reach across the British Isles to the external manifestations of this disorder than we can conclude that the internal illness or disorder cannot be eliminated or cured through the suppression of symptoms than a conflict on the opposite side of the globe can be stopped by securing reports from home.

We should not try to 'cure' or block these signs or symptoms However, with Homeopathy, let us create a healthy environment where our bodies are able to regain their health and symptoms of poor health will vanish.

1.2 What is HOMEOPATHY?

There's a lot to say about "why Homeopathy But what exactly is Homeopathy? As I tried to explain in the previous part, Homeopathy is the reason why a medicine is prescribed as well as the rationale behind prescriptions and not the actual medicine. As an example, as I have mentioned, one could purchase an ounce of Homeopathic tablets from a pharmacy with the name "tablets to treat Lumbago as well as Sciatica'. However, even though the tablets are Homoeopathically manufactured, it isn't Homeopathy since the person is not considered.

In other words, if this is the motive behind giving the medicine essential then what are the motives? The principle of homeopathy may be best described with the Latin phrase: SIMILIA, SIMILIBUS CURRENTUR' which means to allow similar substances to be utilized to treat the same diseases.

What exactly does this mean in the real world? It is the process of taking note of the distinct features of the patient's symptoms and then compare them to known effects of a substance which produces a set of symptoms that are similar to those displayed by the patient. This will be the SIMILIMUM.

Let's illustrate this point A sting from a bee may cause the appearance of a red and flaming swelling that stings and burns and is extremely sensitive the touch, causing pain and stiffness. It feels better in colder temperatures, but more so when it is warm.

It is now time to consider Similimum in the event of an individual suffering from, say such as arthritis in the knee which was affected by oedema (swollen and filled with liquid) white, and smooth extremely sensitized to contact, it hurt and burned, but the one thing that brought relief was cold application but if she stepped close to the fire, the heat would aggravate the problem. and we used Apis. It is a mellifica (honey honey bee sting) and that's because we've taken all signs into account to determine the similimum that would be the right medicine.

What can we do? Find a jar of bees and let them to sting our dear? It's been done and it was done in cases where similimum proper relief was achieved, (Interestingly, an ancient treatment for arthritis was to the open of an nest of ants and allow the insects to sting It appears to have been a similar idea that is demonstrated in this case.) However, there is a better method that you'll be delighted to learn.

The development of Homeopathy began in the time that of Hahnemann, who is the present day pioneer of the principle. studies have been conducted to establish the exact records of the effect of various substances on human beings. The Homeopathic medicine is never tested on animals as, aside of the HUMANE aspect, it would be a an untruth in the homeopathic Principle and therefore the medicines need to be tested on human subjects. This process is known as Proving. Hahnemann himself was the one who conducted a large variety of these tests and this is the way it was carried out by selecting the appropriate volunteers , male and female were chosen, they were required to be healthy and in good shape, with conditions of no stress that might alter the results. They also had to be completely open and open about their perceptions of their own experiences, feelings etc.

The 'provers', or 'provers' as they were known were given doses of remedy. If the remedy was one which normally exerts an effect upon the human body particularly when it was poisonous the small amount was given every day. If it was an inert chemical such as chalk, which is not a significant influence on the human body , the effectiveness of the ingredient was released and made more potent by diluting. Yes! Through the course of trials it was found that more more power could be removed from a substance with the careful diluting process or potentisations, each one being Shaken vigorously or thoroughly (we will discuss the potencies in a bit).

So substances that had minimal or no effect on their natural state became treatments and slowly the records constructed about the impact of remedies on physical, mental and emotional health conditions of the "provers who used them, and after thorough examination of Hahnemann and his colleagues , a complete description of the remedies' properties was compiled and the 'MateriaMedica Pura was created. In addition, if you visit Hahnemann's "Materia the Medica

Pura' it provides the names of long-suffering provers.

To return to our patient with an arthritic knee, we can offer the Apis Mellifica in potency thus following the fundamental rules that are the basis of Homeopathy, SIMILIA, SIMILIBUS, CURRENTUR and the MINIMUM DOSE.

2 CASE TAKENING

This is where the situation into consideration, lies the most important connection leading to the correct solution being discovered, because If the wrong information is used to draw your conclusions, you'll surely come up with an incorrect conclusion.

You might have the most sophisticated and sophisticated computer on the planet that can make the right decisions , but if you put in incorrect information into its memory bank , even though it can provide answers to your queries, the conclusions will be flawed The conclusion will be accurate in the sense that the data is concerned, but it is useless. The old saying goes "rubbish in, rubbish out." So we need to be exact to arrive at an accurate assessment.

The case is taken before any words are spoken, and it is done through OBSERVATION In fact, observation is an essential part of the process. How is the patient seated while waiting? What is their attire and groomed? Pay attention to their the colour of their hair, complexion and weight. Also, the skin's texture and age. Make sure you shake hands. What type of handshake does it give you?

After we have seated us in a comfortable manner, the next step, after determining the name of the patient, their address, age , and the medication currently taken is to let the patient to explain the motive behind their appearance before you with their words and at their own pace and in the arrangement they would like. Some may bring a tidy list of their symptoms (which is, in and of own way, an indication of their personality) however it's better to have them describe their experience to you or use their list to help them remember. This is to show what symptoms pop up in their minds and will also allow you to see how they describe their symptoms naturally.

In this moment, while taking note of the information you're being given be sure to take note of how the patient relay the information in a coherent and way, without rushing or does everything come out in no order, quickly jumping from one topic to the next or is the person unable to speak about anything All of these factors are pertinent and serve as helpful in determining the patient's mental health.

Once he's completed the narrative in the way it naturally occurs from the notes you made, go back and review the information covered by asking questions to open the patient's eyes' bit more. Be wary of questions that might be answered with a no or yes answer. Be aware of this fact: certain people naturally like to please. should you permit the person to know where the question is heading and he will be swept by it to the extent that he'll provide responses that he believes are the right answer to your question and not necessarily what is actually his experience.

Don't let your thoughts be pulled off at the tangent of one treatment too soon because your questions reflect this preconceived notions of yours. You are likely to get only the answers you need to hear, and that match your beliefs. Therefore, try to find the logical route of questions before heading off on the wrong direction or you'll miss crucial questions that could be beneficial, and you'll have to go back to the foundation questions later since the patient is not benefiting from the treatment you given them.

The next step is to find patterns within the symptoms and isolate the most important ones. In order to do this, we divide these symptoms into 3 categories,

Mental Health, GENERALS and PARTICULARS.

When you listen to us, what can we to distinguish between Mentals Generals, Particulars, and Mentals? Mentals, for the most part, are self-explanatory; they represent the mindset or response of the person's response to his or her experiences, his surroundings as well as to other people and to the world, his goals, aspirations, desires and beliefs, as well as religious motives concepts of life quality and so on. The emotions these elements generate within the person.

One method to distinguish general symptoms from specific ones is to pay focus on how they describe their symptoms. If they are using the terms'my" and "me" when they describe a symptom, they subconsciously include the symptom throughout their self. Other expressions like 'there's the feeling of pain or 'foot" are expressions that differentiate the specific symptom from the entire person. It is important to pay attention and pay attention to the underlying cause. A set of unrelated specific symptoms can cause a general symptom. such as:

Although the four symptoms could be described in a different way by the patient, you would be required to look for the common symptoms of left-sidedness in all complaints , and it is more important than the totality of specific symptoms.

General symptoms are common to every person, so for instance all symptoms can appear suddenly or become violent, or they might be burning as a typical symptom. The most common feature among symptoms is a crucial general sign. The whole person might be more comfortable in bed, but the specific symptoms of itching could be more severe when lying in a warm bed. it's more crucial than the specific.

It is crucial to identify TIME modes. If symptoms appear are they accompanied by a time-based cycle? The time-span could occur every 10-15 minutes for acute conditions or each autumn in chronic cases. The duration of the cycle is variable.

The patient should be asked about his medical history as well as that of his family. Often, a chronic condition that is inherited from the past could require treatment before. For instance, he might not have been able to get well from the time he had whooping cough as an infant. What are his thoughts regarding the root reason for the current problem? One of the most insightful one to ask is "What has been your most painful emotional experience in your life? Ask, 'What is your most joy? These questions force the person to reflect on the path the person has traveled on his path to ill health and help them to realize that we reap what we plant'. Many people think that an emotional disturbance is the source of their physical issues However, due to materialism or a deeply trained habit of avoiding emotions, they put these thoughts to one side and look for a physical cure. When you help people to consider the emotional triggers you will be able to establish an atmosphere that a genuine solution is likely to emerge.

Temperature-related modalities are crucial, and as is the aggravation or reduction from extreme heat and cold can be a sign of individual solutions or reactions towards the results of exercise, rest and passive or active movement. Meteorological techniques can be extremely beneficial in their reactions to upcoming thunderstorms and direct sunlight and sea air, for example.

In all of these conversations, observe and, especially with emotional subject, their reactions (For instance, Pulsatilla weeps on relating symptoms, Sepia weeps on being asked) And while some men will stifle his emotions in front of you, you can ask him : What could cause you to weep and cry?' And remember that it's not only the answer that has significance, but also the way you react.

Physical signs like discharges, odours, skin appearance, type, and the nature of pain, and appearance are helpful to determine a "type" i.e. an emaciated, pale sandy haired blue-eyed girl who is easily triggered to tears, especially when sick, and who gets along perfectly with animal pals might require Pulsatilla or a slim, tall delicate, red-haired girl with long eyelashes and elegant manner of speaking, eager to provide the right answers to your queries could require Phosphorus. But these types of images regarding physical appearance are just the pointers but we mustn't overlook that Mentals as well as Generals and Time factors are much more important.

3 MATERIA 3 MATERIA

According to the definition, Materia Medica means the substances employed in medicine: the science behind their properties and their use. A reliable Materia Medica is vital for Homeopathic prescribing. There are a variety of available, including reprints of the original texts of Samuel Hahnemann's "Materia of Medica Pura'. In the years since Hahnemann's writings, other remedies have been "proved and added to the more modern Materia Medicas. They are beneficial for our contemporary society which is subject to increased demands and exposure to toxic substances which are exclusive in the twentieth Century.

133

If you're first beginning with an Materia Medica, the amount of information could seem overwhelming. The common reaction is to just put it all down once more, but do not do this, it's simply an issue of starting by focusing on one thing at each step. While you can find books that provide potted Materia Medica as pointers, you'll feel more content when you understand the reason you're taking a specific remedy. It is therefore important to be aware of a few of the common remedies well , and then expand on the knowledge you have gained.

If you're looking to purchase an Materia Medica may I suggest some classics that you might want to look into for: -

Seminars about Homeopathic Materia Medica J.T. Kent

Homeopathic Drug Pictures Tyler

The leaders in Homeopathic Nash Therapeutics

An Dictionary of Practical Materia Medica 3 volumes of Clarke

There are also brand new contemporary Materia Medicas coming onto the market that include certain of the more rare lesser-used remedies, however a basic set of remedies is sufficient to begin with. These books will provide the complete list of prover's symptoms (see chapter one for an explanation of the purpose that provers play in.) But the abbreviated Materia Medica at the end of this course will assist you get the gist or the main signs of some of the more popular treatments.

You'll notice that I've attempted to outline every treatment in the same manner by separating the key words as a memory aid then the aggravation and the amelioration as well as the mental symptoms and in some cases , the cause. Other symptoms are described under the functions or parts in the body. It is also evident that there are notes for prescribers at the end of each remedy , indicating the compatibility between remedies and any other comments regarding length of time that the remedy is effective.

Chapter 7: Repertory

From the drugs discussed in the previous section, you'll notice that some of these "pictures" as they are described are as intricate as the person who is taking them and that's just how it is supposed to be.

The most effective method to become familiar with the contents the Materia Medica is to take one image of medicine at a time from an organized, well thought down Materia Medica and read it attentively, looking for patterns which run throughout the remedies. For example , bleeding, burning and blindness can be utilized as a way to remember this remedy Phosphorus. If you've found the "spirit" remedy, you can move on to another. By doing this, you will quickly gain an understanding of essential remedies.

If you're faced with unwell child in the past, the pressure of the situation may render all your memories of your schooling disappear in the early hours like mist in the dawn.

This is the reason Kent's Repertory was created (there are other Repertories as well, however Kent's is most well-known and the most well-known for our illustration). A Repertory is a text that lists the symptoms in logical sequence and includes the drugs that exhibit the symptoms. For instance, if a medication causes a specific reaction in test subjects, or people who received the substance to test for, the substance is listed under the symptoms heading in the Repertory.

For example: Kent's Repertory, page 454

Tonsils / THROAT

Cold weather, each and every day of Dulc. and hep.

painless: Bapt.

recurrent: Alumn., Bar-c., bar-m., hep.,

lach., lyc., psor., sang., sep., sil., sulph.

Listings are registered in the following formats: -

1. Normal type

2. Italics

3. Bold

to emphasize the significance of the symptom, or how it is a characteristic in the context of that specific medicine.

The symptoms are as follows There are symptoms to look for:

1. Part of the body

2. Condition

3. General

4. Particular

For instance:

1. Chest

2. Pain

3. Motion aggravates

4. Of the arms

So, symptoms that concern the entire of a person (Generals) have precedence over those relating to a particular part (Particulars). I am unable to do much better than to take a line from the introduction of Kent's Repertory on the best way to utilize the book:

After taking the case in accordance with the rules laid out by the Organon (see chapter on case taking) take note of every mental symptom and any symptoms or conditions that are that are attributed to the patient and then search the patient's repertory for signs that are similar to the above. Look for physical signs that are based on the colour by the colour of blood, of discharge, and body discomfort and improvement that affects the entire body, and also craving for fresh air, a desire for warmth or cold air, to rest or movement, which could be merely a desire, or may cause the feeling of general improvement. It is important to understand that a situation which causes the whole body to feel more or less well is much more significant as compared to a situation that is only affecting the part that is painful or the part that is completely different. You can further personalize it with the symptom-based explanations derived from functioning, organs and feelings and always assigning a crucial location to the moment of the onset of each sign until each aspect is scrutinised. Examine the symptoms together, in comparison and individually and then study your Materia Medica of such remedy or remedies that run through the symptoms of the condition to make sure there's no question the one that is most like among all treatments.'

Therefore, we're requested to identify all symptoms and their causes (that that cause the symptoms to become better or worse, or any other concomitant (accompanying) signs that are associated in conjunction with the complaint) Write them down in order of importance i.e. Generals, Mentals Particulars, and search them in the literature. List the drugs under the symptoms that are relevant Read and compare the pictures of medicines within the Materia Medica and decide which is the closest.

Repertory is an extremely precise method of comparing symptoms with remedies however, the recording of all the medications even in their abbreviated form , is extremely laborious and this is where the repertorisation sheets come into.

A repertorisation worksheet lists 255 names of medicines, that are alphabetical. On top of that are 11 columns. At the very top, create an important rubric (symptom) which you write again according to importance, and using the repertory, label the box with the treatment that the symptom requires is identified with a 1, 2 or 3 based on the level of stress given to the symptoms from the repertory. Continue to do this for each symptom until it will be apparent that a pattern has emerged. There are a few medications or perhaps only one will be recommended however, it's not enough to take the'score' on the repertorisation form, you have to go over the Materia Medica and compare the entire list before selecting the treatment.

POTENCY AND REPETITION

5.1 Which is the potency?

As he compiled notes about the responses of "provers" to medicines and substances Hahnemann discovered that an inert chemical can cause an effect on a person when it is diminished (potentised) and pounded or shaken.

The more tests proved that the higher the "dilution the more deeply the drug was able to work as well as the stronger it was. This is how the term "potency" was coined'.

Typically, the term "potency" refers to two scales: the decimal scale, 1 part in 10 and the Centesimal 1 part in 100. The decimal scale is denoted by an "X" (i.e. Arnica 6x) and the Centesimal by the letter 'C' (i.e. Arnica 30c) or in the United Kingdom a number on its own with no suffix is considered to be Centesimal (i.e. Arnica 30).

In the preparation of the medicines it is necessary to use a single component, i.e. 1 mg, of the base substance, for instance we're creating Natrum Muriaticum - the substance will be common salt and TEN components, i.e. 10 mg of the base substance (in this case , water or alcohol) The two are then vigorously shaken or succussed in a symbiosis. Some pharmacies continue to use this method by hand, literally hitting the bottle against the book to trigger the sucussion. This has led to the development of 1X. This action is the basis principle of vibration, or active force, or whatever you wish to call is released from an impermeable substance (the salt) and is picked in by the basic substance.

Now, we take one portion of our 1X , mix it with 10 parts of base substance , and then make a succuss, thereby making 2X.

In the event of an insoluble material such as a metal, then the first three dilutes are made through trituration or grinding with the mortar and pestle along with milk sugar as the basis substance. After the third time of trituration, ANY substance becomes soluble and is able to be made potent by the process that was described earlier. The process of dilution in series is repeated until the desired amount of potency has been achieved. The same procedure is followed when making the Centesimal range, but the ratio for the steps is one 100.

What exactly is "the desired potency the desired potency'? How do I determine what potency I should use? Potency is not a misnomer as this process. It is able to release power. The higher the power, the more fine the power. Therefore, we need to make sure the power is compatible with the task to be completed. It is not necessary to break an egg using the sledgehammer.

We are multi-faceted creatures that are driven by a deep and an active force, which is the emotional and spiritual aspects that, in a deeper way, controls the functioning in our body. For instance, a person could stay warm all winter long and not be sick, only to succumb to illness after a few days later after experiencing a devastating emotional or physical shock. I'm sure you'll be able to think of instances where this happened to you.

This is due to being able to say that our control of emotions was impacted and has physical effects. We choose our arsenal depending on our goals. If we're dealing with the earth , earthy and by this, I'd include symptoms as well as a kind of person, then we should use the lower or 'X' potencies. In contrast, when a physiological issue had its roots, or is causing of an emotional disturbance or if the individual is an extremely "arty" emotional type , then a higher capacity, such as the "C" range might be needed.

High potencies are great for acute situations, however it is recommended to go with a lower dose for chronically long-term illness.

The above can be illustrated in a case I dealt with a few years back. A man was referred to me with an horrific anal fistula. He was treated by some of the world's most renowned Doctors and underwent surgeries several times, but the painful and uncomfortable condition recurred each time. This meant that it was impossible for him in his work place for variety of years.

When I asked him about it, he said that his condition was a result of after his dad's death. I wasn't, however, having to deal with a simple case of griefthat would be a good reason to have Ignatia as well Nat. Mur. It appears that this man lived right next to his father who was dying and was a great help to the man in his final days. His brother was in town and would stop by each night on his return home from work to visit his father, who eagerly anticipated the time of visit. My patient was irritated for a long time over what he perceived to be the unfairness of the situation, however because he was afraid to provoke a reaction in the last days of his father's life, the patient bottled up his frustration. When I inquired if he'd ever talked to his brother since but he replied that since his father was gone, and he didn't have any additional burden of doing therefore what was the point.

Staphisagria is the most effective cure for suppressed anger - one pilule of 200th centesimal power led to the most complete and long-lasting cure.

5.2 Do you use it often?

There is a basic guideline to follow when prescribing. It is to wait until the first dose take effect before giving any more as this is the case equally to chronic and acute ailments. A child suffering from acute symptoms that require Belladonna might be immediately relieved with the first dose, however, that relief could be brief before a second dose is needed which could last some time before the next dose is required for repeated. In contrast, one dose of a medication for an ongoing condition can provide relief that lasts for weeks or even months.

In the past, If a remedy that is Homeopathic does not work, it's not the medicine's fault and the blame lies somewhere else; let us discuss that claim.

If we do not experience any reaction to a medication, it could be due to:

1. We gave the wrong remedy, or the wrong dosage and ...

2. It is a slow-acting remedy.

3. That the patient is slow in his response and has diminished vitality, and the disease is becoming fatal in its direction. Therefore, we need to reevaluate the situation.

There are three or four excellent reactions we can obtain These are: -

1. A solid, gradual improvement that didn't cause any discomfort. This indicates that we were right on. Do not continue to give medicine.

2. A brief sharp aggravation, then a steady improvement. This is a great thing. Patients who suffer from this initial discomfort usually recover very well. There is no further medication until it is called for.

3. Improvement of symptoms , followed by a temporary returning of symptoms from the Past, returning in reverse order in which they first appeared. This is beneficial the following reasons, as per Herrings Law:

"All cure begins from the inside out, head to foot and in reverse order once the symptoms appear in the past! Don't give any advice an answer, as the symptoms of the past is usually gone by itself, but when they do, identify them as the most important signs to help you complete the treatment.

4. A long-term aggravation, with slow improvement. It's a difficult thing to manage, but it is necessary to be patient, your body is evidently low in energy and we have to be patient and allow it to go as it pleases, we have an extremely weak system.

If, despite a given treatment, the body does not be able to respond and instead it gradually and slowly declines, then there is nothing we can do but reduce the symptoms and, in turn, ensure that the patient is as comfortable as is possible.

HAHNEMANN AND THE SPIRIT Like DYNAMIS

Samuel Hahnemann, in his book "Organon of Medicine" The basis of his approach is on the concept of a spirit-like energy that exists through the physical body. Every bodily function, feeling and sensation. is influenced and experienced by the energy of dynamism. The body's physical form is then animated through the force of spirit which utilizes the body as an instrument or tool. (Organon 9,10,15,16.)

Hahnemann is here to reveal his evidently Christian roots and influences. If we look at the official views of the church of the time (which views continue to this day) there is a common conviction that the soul is immortal. Therefore, it is not surprising for him to imagine a spirit-like force "living within' our bodies. Without this force we wouldn't be.

The Dogma of the eternality of the soul is different between religions, but the basic principles are:

1. A soul is a part of a person inside him, and is not a any part of him.

2. The soul is immortaland unending.

3. The soul is released from its body on the moment of death and resurfaces in a spirit body.

He was able to see that there was a vital force' that exists in every living person or an 'life principle' or 'principle of living' and this alone is proof of the genius of Hahnemann. He understood that force is what gives people willpower or personality is a natural occurrence because of the teachings of the Church that were prevalent at the time.

Let's take a review of the spiritual dynamism (vital power) that Hahnemann's Organon 15 theory in the context of the largest read book in the history of mankind and that's the Bible. I'm sure that Hahnemann would have been pleased.

We must first understand the meaning of four terms from Hebrew as well as Greek (the language of both the Old and New Testament).

HEBREW GREEK MEANING IN ENGLISH

Chai-yim' Zo-e' Life principle

Ru'ach Pneu'ma Life force (spirit)

Ne'phesh's Psy-khe's The Life of an Soul

Nesha-mah' Pno-e' Life sustaining breath

We will now look at some of the references in the Authorized King James Bible and look at the different meanings of terms are employed:

Genesis verse 7

"And The LORD God created man from dirt from the earth breathing into his nostrils life-giving breath (Nesha-mah" Chai-yim') and man became an eternal spirit (Ne'phesh). "

We are aware that Hahnemann was right when he said that the body composed of chemical constituents is not a soul that is in existence until made to live through the introduction of the life principle (Chai-yim') and the "sustaining breath" (Nesha-mah') to keep the process going.

However , in Organon 15 Organon 15 we find him declaring:

"The organism is in fact the physical instrument of living, but it's impossible to imagine without the motion given to it by ability to sense and regulate dynamism and vital force can't be understood in the absence of an organism. Therefore, the two elements together form one." (So so far, so good. the Genesis account stated that it needed the principle of life (Chai-yim') and sustaining breath (Nesha-mah') to make the body live).

To continue -

"Although in thought , our mind divides this oneness into two distinct notions in order to make it easier for understanding."

What is the reason we separate them for ease of understanding"? Because in our minds is the concept of a spiritual component within us which is different and has a purpose and continues to exist beyond the death of the body.

Let us be clear, when God created the first human being, Adam He created his body from the 'dust from the ground or the elements, and then infused into every tissue of your body the concept of life. This meant that the man lived and 'became a soul living' (note he did not have a soul implanted in the first place, but he was born with one) and then God initiated the man's breathing to sustain and maintain the existence. So a person can only endure for a few minutes without breathing before the life principle starts to die , and it is those brain cells, first. This life principle isn't USING our body to perform any function. But what is the life force, or spirit (Ru'ach Pneu'ma) is it residing in us? Let us go back to our previous example to gain a better understanding:

Ecclesiastes verse

"For what befalls the children of men, it also befalls beasts, and a single thing happens to them. If one dies and dies, the other also dies as well. They are the same breath (Ru'ach the word for life force, or spirit) to the point that a human does not have any preeminence over beasts: because everything has a price." Authorized King James Bible

It is evident in this passage it is true that the energy, or spirit that powers humans is identical to that which stimulates animals. What is more, when the animal or man dies, the Ru'ach, the life force or spirit, is gone. The spirit, or the active force can be compared to a different invisible force - electricity, which despite being a non-person, it can enable machines to play music or travel, calculate mathematical equations , etc. And when the machine is turned off the source of power ceases to flow.

In actual William Boericke in his footnotes to the Organon appreciates the dynamic influence of magnetism as a comparable force. It is not the spirit or life principle can live inside the body with a will to make use of our physical bodies.

While not possessing willpower or personality In the end, the Life Force, or as Hahnemann calls it"the Dynamis is the word that refers to health and life. Any disruption could be a huge impact on our physical and mental health.

How content Samuel Hahnemann would have been to have a complete knowledge of the essential forces within our bodies and affecting us in both sickness as well as in health.

We believe that having an understanding the benefits Homeopathic prescribing will improve the wellbeing and well-being of your entire family for years to be.

Chapter 8: The Way To Identify A Disease

Hahnemann presented the specifics of this revolutionary method of medicine in 1810 in a work titled The Organon der Heilkunst or Organon of the Remedial Art. The work is commonly called simply the Organon.

The German term employed in the work of Dr. Hahnemann, Heilkunst, describes the two aspects of healing and the removal of the disease.

The English word "remediation" (to remediate or rectify) best describes the two components of Heilkunst. This is why the word "remedy" is often used to describe the use of medicines to treat ailments based on laws of similarities or what is generally referred to as "homeopathic remedies'.

Heilkunst, also known as healing, or the practice of returning health Healthcare includes both the use of drugs to eliminate disease, as well as healing, or aiding the ability of the body to restore the system back to normal after the illness has been eliminated.

in the Introduction to the 1st version of the Organon, Hahnemann made clear that he was creating an entirely revolutionary system of medical treatment to treat diseases that was totally at contrast to the current systems of treatment, and that his method was backed through careful observation and experimentation:

Through this inquiry, I discovered the way to truth that I am required to walk on my own, a path that is far from the typical path of the medical routine. The further I moved away towards truth and the more my conclusions depart from the old structure that was based on the assumption of opinions, was supported solely by opinion, however I refused to allow any of my opinions to be held until they were confirmed through experimentation. The outcomes of my convictions are presented within this publication.

Hahnemann's main concern was on the elimination of diseases. In his epigrammatic style, he spells the issue precisely in the very first three aphorisms in his most famous work known as the Organon.

The job of a medical professional is

To be aware of how to spot disease(s).

to understand the curative potential of every medicinal ingredient

to treat each illness with a similar treatment

Understanding the nature of the disease process is therefore extremely important. However, before we look at the question "What does it mean to be a the definition of disease?" we need to examine the two methods Hahnemann offers us in the treatment of diseases.

Two Disease Categories

The doctor. Hahnemann determined that there were two different types of diseases that required a different approach to using laws of similarities.

* primary illnesses that had the same essence or nature,

* secondary illnesses that evolved from primary diseases and were of a varied nature.

Chronic or Tonic Diseases

The most common diseases can be recognized by their distinctive symptoms, but also due to their usual cause that is well-known like an accident, a poisoning, or any other obvious trauma to the body. Since these conditions are the most crucial and essential and fundamental, they are of paramount importance to Dr. Hahnemann often referred to them as affecting the sound or tone of an individual's well-being, which is why they are referred to as 'tonic' illnesses.

The first examples of these illnesses were the self-limiting diseases of childhood, including myasles, scarlet fever and measles (these are later identified as disease pathogenic) and trauma-related injury (e.g., bruises, falls, or emotional shocks which Hahnemann described as homogenous in the nature of things). Hahnemann also included Iatrogenic or drug-induced illnesses.

Hahnemann realized that there was a single solution for each of the permanent, fixed ailments. The exact remedy for every chronic disease was simple to determine by using common law as a reference. The majority of the treatments to be used in first-aid scenarios are to treat chronic illnesses, such as Arnica Montana to treat bruises or contusion diseases.

Pathologic or Variable Diseases

Secondary diseases are harder to recognize especially when they arise by a primary or a tonic illness. In most cases, treating for a tonic illness will cure secondary diseases that are related and, in some cases, these illnesses remain unaffected and require to be treated with the same medication. As an example, if you treat for a serious case of chickenpox using the particular regular - in this instance a remedy known as Varicella that eliminates the main tonic disease chickenpox, a few significant signs might remain. These, are examined and show a secondary illness caused by the virus itself. The symptom image is associated with an identical symptom picture created by a remedy used in healthy people and, then, through an act of similarity, this secondary illness is also eliminated.

The relationship between the two is then determined based on the manifestation of symptoms and the "pathology" that is the disease within the patient. And, therefore, these illnesses are also known as "pathological" diseases.

In some cases, especially complicated chronic conditions that are not clear, there is no root cause or the cause is multiple and would require some time to treat these ailments. These types of cases are the mainstay of diseases that are currently. Since they stem from the primary disease and cannot be distinguished in relation to the their cause, but instead upon the symptoms that each illness exhibits, which manifest primarily through changes in emotions of functions, sensations, and feelings.

Treatment based solely on symptoms isn't an easy task when the problem is a long-lasting one. The treatment that was employed for one instance of headache, for instance, is not always the case in the following case since the primary illnesses can lead to various secondary ailments every time. So, there is no cure for headaches or indigestion, because the causes of secondary illnesses that cause headaches or indigestion could differ depending on the particular case.

The pathological method can be useful when the condition is severe and the symptoms are clear, which is typically the case in the context of home-care or first-aid.

The Order of Disease Treatment

In this regard, Hahnemann realized that the first step is to recognize the primary, constant ailments. Once this is accomplished it is possible to have the treatment easily identified. The treatment that comprises the bulk of first-aid treatments is fast, effective and efficient treatment by using a variety of remedies found in a homeopathic first-aid kit of remedies (information about how to get one of them is provided at the at the end in the text).

True Disease and False Disease

The Dr. Hahnemann attacked the prevailing perception of illness as it misinterpreted the effects of illness (mostly symptoms and signs) as either the disease itself, or worse it was the causes of the disease. This is the current situation. So, a patient is diagnosed with bowel inflammation and is assumed to be the result of the disease in itself and referred to as irritable colon disease'. This is because the illness is thought of as which can be eliminated with medications (anti-inflammatories in this instance) or eliminated through surgery if it becomes severe enough.

For Hahnemann The symptoms do not reflect the disease however, they are the manifestation.

It is necessary to look deeper to discover the alteration of the vital force that causes the symptoms we refer to as symptoms. For primary illnesses, this involves identifying the cause or the agent that causes the disorder - - whether it's an emotional trauma, accident or microbe, as well as poison (including medications).

Fortunately, in the majority of cases of first-aid, the root causes are easily identifiable: an insect bite, burn, cut or scratch or scratch, etc. And for every cause, there's a remedy specific to the cause for each, like Arnica Montana for any injury that is a physical hit to the body, which is usually characterized by bruises ('contusion condition').

Arnica montana gives healthy individuals the sensation as it was if they were hit or beat (bruised sensation) and, therefore due to its law of analogies eliminates the trauma of the physical impact it allows for the body to heal the injury. Although the body can recover from the contusion, but without getting rid of the disease that caused it however, it can create a feeling of feeling of weakness, discomfort or pain until the disease is eliminated. The body can heal itself from any wound but the marks remain as evidence that the disease isn't gone. You might know someone who suffers from the weakness, limitation, or pain continues to persist even after an accident like whiplash or a serious sprain ankle is a result. Another indication of a residual injury to our body can be seen in the appearance of a wound. If the condition is correctly eliminated and healed, the body can then complete the process of restoring health. There are no scars or lingering pains. There will be no limitations in movement, or the weak spots that persist.

The Dr. Hahnemann also criticized the tendency to focus on an atypical symptom like diarrhea and to overlook the specific, individual signs of each individual case and ensure that there was no way that two cases of irritable bowel are necessarily identical.

Therefore, if one incident of irritable bowel syndrome was brought on by an emotional trauma , and another was caused by a microbial infection the treatment would be different for each , based on the root of the problem being different. Additionally, if one patient was suffering from bowel irritation that was relieved by eating, and the other was more irritable due to eating, then each will require treatment differently.

Very little useful information from the conventional Methods

So, as per the doctor Dr. Hahnemann, no truly relevant medical information can be derived from the standard method (which is basically identical today as it was) due to two reasons:

* A sign or symptom is not the actual disease and naming it like colitis or arthritis doesn't transform the effects of the illness.

* Unless the more personalizing symptoms and symptoms of disease in the patient are taken into consideration also, it's impossible to determine the illness.

As Hahnemann advised, specific treatments for illness can only be discovered when the root cause of disease was discovered.

Summary of the Principles

As of now, you've been taught:

1. It is a dynamic disease and requires a continuously active medicine. The symptoms we feel or observe in the body are the result an imbalance in the energy body, which is what drives it. The mental and physical effects of the disturbances can be diminished through diet, nutrition, relaxation as well as loving care. However, the root of the disease

is only able to be eliminated through a homeopathic remedy.

2. A cure's law is the one of similarities. In other words, you need to provide a remedy that can create in a healthy person the same disease as that for the person suffering. So, if the patient is suffering from symptoms similar to those of poisoning due to Deadly Nightshade (Belladonna) However, they have never eaten anything from the herb, giving a dilute dose of Belladonna that is prepared homeopathically will cure the illness in the patient.

3. There are two kinds of illnesses: those that have a variable nature, and are referred to as pathological and those that remain constant in nature, which are referred to as tonic. Pathological diseases need to be identified by examining the symptoms that are caused by the disease and then finding a cure which is similar to the picture of the disease. Tonic illnesses are diagnosed easier, often by the reason like the impact of an instrument that is blunt, resulting in bruise (which requires Arnica montana or Mountain Laurel).

4. The most frequent, tonic illnesses are those we see in first-aid (bruises or sprains bones, concussions, burns as well as insect bites, poisoning from food, etc.) as well as in the basic infections of childhood, like chickenpox, whooping cough, as well as other outbreaks.

The pathological, variable illnesses are those we encounter in varied conditions, such as headaches, colds and flus and allergy symptoms digestion issues, etc.

Dose and Potency for First Aid and home use

In general, in urgent or first-aid situations, you'll:

1. Utilize whatever potency you have available (6C 12, 12C, 30,, and 200C are commonly used in remedy kits). More potent remedies work better for more urgent situations.

2. Repeat the dose frequently the more severe (acute) the condition.

3. An approach that is common in circumstances where you are likely to need to take multiple doses it to dissolve a couple of tiny pellets or a drop of the remedy in stock in

approximately 4 oz or 125 milliliters of water (preferably bottle-sealed) and then stir it vigorously for several times or move it around in your palm for about a couple of minutes. Then, you can drink a glass of this solution as a single dose.

4. The frequency can vary from a couple of seconds, in severe circumstances such as anaphylactic shock. every few minutes during high fever, or within 15-30 minutes during the majority of instances.

5. The better the patient's experience more comfortable, the less often you'll need to repeat the procedure.

Further details on the method of creating potent and dynamized remedies, as well as the numbers, like 6x, 12D and 30C and 30CH, refer to are available in the chapter dedicated to Homeopathic Pharmacy.

Fundamental Principles to Choose the Best Treatment

Tonic First

The first, and preferred method of medicine is to determine the root of the problem.

In homeopathic medicine, this method is known as continuous or tonic prescribing, instantly provides you with the treatment is needed to get rid of the cause of the condition (and to treat the symptoms or the condition that are that are caused by the reason). This is according to the doctor Dr. Hahnemann stated, true causal prescribing.

In most instances the tonic method will suffice and is the one you should initially try to employ.

The Pathic If Not

In some instances the primary, or tonic illness may be the cause of an additional, pathological disease. This secondary illness is the result of the primary disease in the circumstances of the patient's particular constitution.

In some general ailments such as colds or headaches, it's not always easy to determine which is the primary cause so you will need to look at the symptoms that are acute to determine the best treatment for your particular instance of a headache or cold.

This leads us to the second method of treating which is known as prescription for pathology. In lieu of being able determine the reason for the disease, the doctor must be able to identify the disease by way specific symptoms that the disease manifests within the patient. This is why the term "pathic prescribing" was coined (symptoms means suffering, which is "pathos" from Greek).

Dual Prescription

There may be situations in which you have to prescribe both tonic as well as the pathological illnesses in a patient with an ailment. You can give each one separately, or offer both remedies simultaneously when you are able to identify the two diseases. This is known as 'dual treatment prescribing'. If the pathological disease is severe there is a good chance that it'll need to be treated, even if you are treating for the tonic disease that causes it.

Let's look at an easy illustration.

Children are exposed to measles. Measles is a recurring tonic disease that is that is of infectious (pathogenic) cause. When it is determined that measles has been diagnosed has been confirmed, the treatment that is Morbillinum is available and administered effectively, and even pre-emptively (see the section dedicated to Prevention).

It is possible that the primary illness develops a secondary type, which then becomes a condition by itself. The severity of this will differ from child to child , and is only discovered by looking at the specific signs and symptoms present in the children. Due to the severity of infectious diseases the degree of variation in secondary or pathological illnesses is largely undefined.

So, typically, there are only a handful of main treatments that can be utilized and the decision can be determined by an easy differential diagnosis that is based on the distinct manifestations of the disease in the patient.

As you will see, the tonic method of prescribing demands the investigation of the underlying causes of the disease as well as understanding of the continuous connection between a particular permanent nature-based illness and the remedy for the disease. The basis for this is the concept established by Dr. Hahnemann from close observation and the clinical experience that "...a permanent or fixed disease requires a permanent or fixed treatment."

However the pathological method of prescribing demands an examination of the symptoms of the disease in relation to the entire spectrum of symptoms for a particular patient. While every diseases have a root however, it's impossible to identify the root cause, which can be the cause of disorder and then take care of what is apparent in the eyes of the patient, which is the pathological disease. You can observe that expression of the pathological disease can differ in patients, even when the tonic disease which is the cause of the disease is identical. It is evident that when we prescribe pathology, we're dealing with the actual disease that causes the symptoms (disease expression , such as irritation, thirst, fever and so on.) by utilizing an individual images or pictures of symptoms rather than simply using a handful of symptoms and suppressing them with an anti-drug as is the standard approach like taking temperature as an overall symptom , and combat it with anti-inflammatory medications (Aspirin, Tylenol, Ibuprofen and so on.)

Find the Solution to simple Trauma

The treatment offered in this field relies on the notion that the scenarios you'll likely encounter are similar for all. Therefore, the treatment for every situation will be the same for every person who is affected by that particular situation (this is known as the law of similarity in the context of the tonic or underlying condition). This makes deciding on the best remedy quite simple after you know what remedies work best for a specific circumstance.

Tonic traumatic illnesses are a part of multiple jurisdictions, as you could have in any country, including a state, federal, and municipal area. The one we'll be focusing upon is homogenic area because the majority of problems involving first-aid stem from this area.

Homogeneous: involving traumas of either a physical or emotional nature that include things like injuries, bee stings sunburn, scrapes, cuts and bruises on the physical side as well as emotional traumas (involving typical traumas within the four categories of anxiety/fear grieving/loss, anger/resentment guilt/jealousy).

It can be a bit odd to view physical manifestations as a form of disease. As you've witnessed, involves an negative change or impingement on the generative aspect of the Living Power. For physical injuries you encounter while prescribing first aid the illness is usually manifested as damage, not an infection or a dynamic affection instead of an active infection. It is possible to believe that our healing power (the sustentive aspect of living Power) is able to recover from injuries, which is the case, however you must be aware the impact on the power of generative persists. This isn't a matter of our healing powers. It can only be treated through medicine based on the principles that the laws of similar resonance are in place.

When we are involved in an accident that is traumatic, like concussions or whiplash it will heal but there will be the feeling of being unwell or of not being fully which we refer to as the "never felt better for a while" feeling. This is caused by the degeneration of the power of regeneration that we experience. This feeling is eliminated from our living power by the correct medication, and restores us to our original condition of health.

The variety of reasons for accidents is quite limited and therefore, the range of options available to deal with these circumstances is also limited and can be learned quickly.

A variety of symptoms or ailments that sufferers are suffering from result from an ongoing trauma or stress. A relationship that is abusive in the workplace in school, at home, or at work can cause us to be traumatized until it results in symptoms like stomachaches, rashes, headaches digestion issues, etc. These are easily and quickly managed if they're fairly recent in origin (they are also treatable even if they've been present in the distant past, and have a negative impact on the health of the patient now but it requires an thorough knowledge about the practice of homeopathy (see the section on the Resources section near the bottom of this article for further details about the process of training to become a homeopath).

Single Traumatic Diseases

Below, you will find the most commonly known causes of a single disease along with their particular (tonic) solutions. These conditions are generally named by the medication utilized to treat them.

Traumas to the body, concussions

Arnica disease

Arnica montana can be described as the main treatment for muscle and bruises and muscle damage, which is which is what Hahnemann described as "contusion condition." This could occur anytime there's physical injuries caused by an injury that is blunt, or from any physical assault on a human body. The signs are muscle soreness, pain, swelling and bruising, and Arnica can quickly heal the signs. It is often the first remedy that people are taught about and utilize as the first treatment that is able to win hearts when they start to recognize the benefits of homeopathic remedies.

177

Arnica can be utilized when individuals are "weekend warriors" who are over-exerting themselves in pursuits that they aren't familiar with. This could happen when one is too busy gardening in the Spring, plays an activity more vigorously than their body is ready for, or is involved in been involved in an accident that causes physical injuries to the body.

Although all of these are physical however, they have caused destruction of the power of generative and this damage must to be addressed. Most people are more inclined to let their body heal itself however, this does not eliminate the shock experienced by the power of generative. This could result in a persistent feeling of malaise. Even though the incident may not have been a significant one but the cumulative impact of these traumas to the body does cost money.

Stresses or traumas to the system regardless of whether they are mental, physical or emotional, can accumulate over time , causing an adverse impact on your life's energy. Imagine a glass of drinking water.

Each incident in your life that affects your ability to generate energy will add a drop of water to the glass. As time passes your glass will begin to overflow. In most cases, we believe where we attribute the latest overflow for the problem however the reality is , the glass needed to be filled before it filled up! Utilizing the right tonic remedies will eliminate any drops that fall from your glass each drop at a and using the right tonic remedy at the time of an event is sure to ensure that the drop does not get being added back to the glass in any way.

According to Clarke's Dictionary of Practical Materia Medica Clarke writes about Arnica:

Arnica is a mountain plant. Arnica is believed to have a natural affinity to the consequences of falling.

According to the German title, Γallkraut, attests, its significance as a vulnerary is in the past since ancient times.

It is described as the trauma most effective.

The trauma of all forms and manifestations, both current and distant can be treated with Arnica like no other drug. these tests demonstrate the effectiveness of the remedy in the symptoms it triggers.

Arnica is an herb that can be consumed internally as powder, granule, or pellet. Arnica can also be found in creams, lotions and oils to be applied externally on the area of contusion.

Note: Arnica is available also in a cream form, however it shouldn't be applied on the outside of a area with damaged skin because Arnica could cause a large amount of irritation in these instances.

Burns

Urtica urensis is a disease

Urtica urens, also known as The Stinging Nettle plant is a treatment that is used to treat minor burns such as sunburns, in which the skin's red as well as a feeling of pain and heat, as well as for scalds caused by hot water. The area that is burned may be soothed by cold application.

Tips: If you suffer a minor burn caused by hot water or another sources of heat, you can utilize to apply the Law of Similars even if you don't carry your homeopathic remedies on hand. The most effective method is to gradually reintroduce the burning to a heat source which caused the initial burn.

It is essential that the heat isn't identical to the intensity which caused the burn, however, it should be similar (in the sense of being less intensive). The pain can be more intense initially, but as you remove the burn from the heat, it will begin to diminish and it will heal in a short time. As the burn's pain increases, you need to lower your heat used.

as Constantine Hering, a famous 19th Century homeopathic doctor, wrote in the homeopathic domestic physician:

Burns and scorches and

In case of a mild burn or scald, the most effective treatment is to hold the area to the flame and then place it in cold water, or apply cooling substances, like turnips, carrots, potatoes or other vegetables. It is well-known that following the blisters, and ulcers are always the result. The former, on contrary is able to draw the heat out which means the burn's effects are eliminated by applying moderate heat. Dry heat however, isn't ever feasible, especially in cases where the burned or scalded area is huge such as this one. the heat is not able to be evenly distributed to each area. For children , the procedure is not a good idea because it is painful. for burns in which the skin has been destroyed or if the wound is on the face, it's not suitable. Alternative treatments, therefore, are required for those who are easier to use, and results are similar to heating.

If the burn is in any way significant the patient must be covered with blankets, then placed next to the fire. Warm water and brandy should be offered. When the warmth has returned, special attention is required to the burned areas.

Cantharis disease

If the burn is more severe that has blisters and damage to the tissue such as in third or second-degree burns, the treatment to consider is Cantharis vesicatoria or Spanish fly. If it is administered quickly enough for chemical burns, even they can help prevent blisters.

Conclusion

Homeopathy gives you the power to improve your overall health and alleviate all ailments you could be suffering from , without relying on costly procedures or hazardous drugs. Utilizing small doses of diluted remedies the practitioners of Homeopathy give patients the ability to conquer ailments by treating the entire person and not just the symptoms. Instead of simply trying to mask the issue like many prescription drugs use today the Homeopathic remedy gets at the root of the issue and offer patients solutions to chronic and acute ailments.

If you're experiencing health issues and are looking for a different approach to conventional treatment and treatments, then Homeopathy might be the perfect option. All you need to enjoy the wide range of advantages that Homeopathic remedies provide are an open-minded mind as well as a fundamental knowledge of Homeopathic principles. It's not just a matter of giving you the power to boost your overall health however, it could also give you the power to conquer any obstacle which may stand between you and an increased level of living.

I hope this Book provides you with the necessary information to start experiencing the numerous advantages that Homeopathy could provide you. Keep in mind that although Homeopathy isn't a panacea and should be used as a component of your overall treatment program, it has the ability to improve your physical, mental and emotional well-being. If it is used correctly it can allow you live a healthy, long-lasting life, without the need for possibly harmful substances.

www.ingramcontent.com/pod-product-compliance
Lightning Source LLC
Chambersburg PA
CBHW060329030426
42336CB00011B/1261